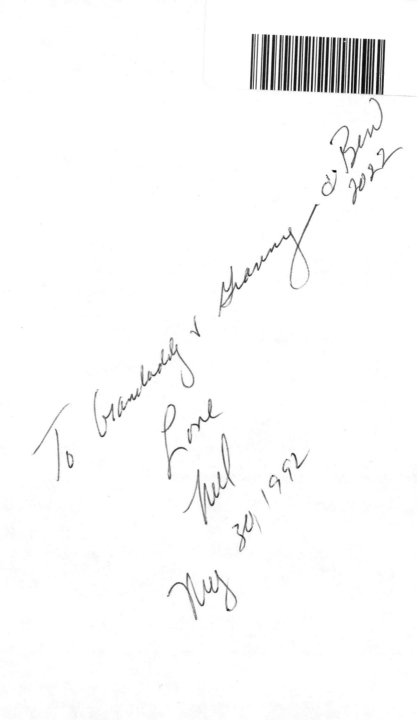

To Grandaddy & Granny & Ben
2022

Love
Neil
30, 1992

Meg

THE GOOD LOOK BOOK

THE GOOD LOOK BOOK

TODAY'S OPTIONS FOR
PROLONGING THE PRIME OF LIFE

Melvin L. Elson, M.D. ▪ John H. Hartley, Jr., M.D.

with Elizabeth Addison

LONGSTREET PRESS
Atlanta, Georgia

Published by
LONGSTREET PRESS, INC.
2140 Newmarket Parkway
Suite 118
Marietta, GA 30067

Printed in the United States of America

1st printing 1992

Library of Congress Catalog Card Number: 91-77191

ISBN 1-5632-029-X

This book was printed by Arcata Graphics, Kingsport, Tennessee. The text was set in Galliard by Laurie Shock.

Cover design by Jill Dible
Cover photo by G. Paul Haynes
Book design by Laurie Shock

This is a work of nonfiction which does not constitute medical advice. Readers should consult with qualified health professionals about their particular needs.

With the exception of specific cases for which the consent of the individual has been obtained, the subjects and patient histories in this work have been partially recounted and changed or combined to protect confidentiality. Names, backgrounds, and places are used fictitiously. The descriptions of actual incidents have also been varied to conceal the identities of those persons involved. Any resemblance to actual events or locales or persons, living or dead, is entirely coincidental.

This book is dedicated to those who will be inspired by its message and who will put the appropriate information to work in order to prolong the prime of their lives and look and feel their very best.

CONTENTS

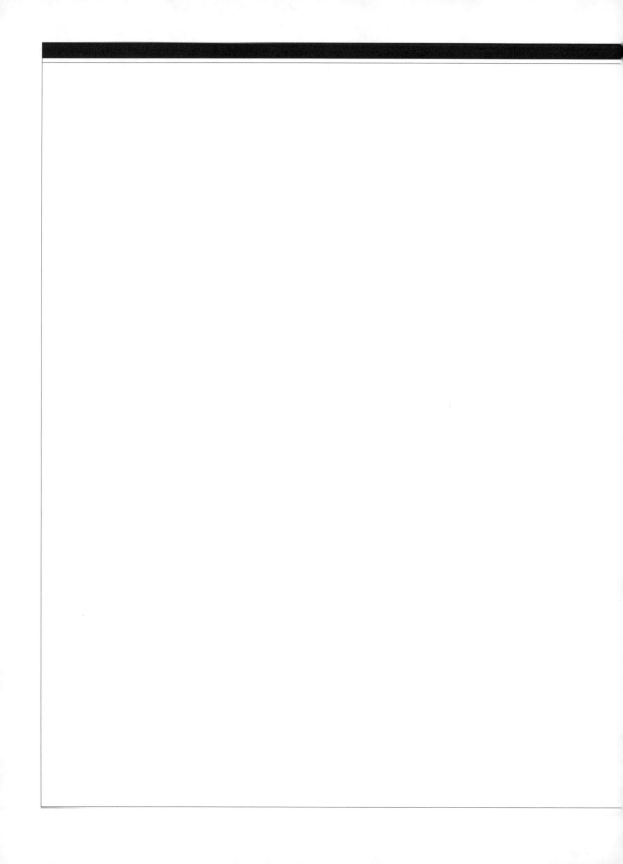

Acknowledgments

We acknowledge the generous assistance and helpful guidance from Suzanne Comer Bell, Marianne Daniels Garber, Ph.D., Ruth J. Norfleet, Barbara Obrentz, and Robyn Freedman Spizman, whose encouragement and expertise helped make *The Good Look Book* a reality. It has been a pleasure to work with Chuck Perry, Caroline Harkleroad, and the entire Longstreet Press staff, whose vision and support have been invaluable. We are also grateful to our families and staff members, who have supported us and contributed to the quality of our lives, and to our patients, who have enabled us to learn from them on a daily basis.

TAKE A GOOD LOOK

> *Life well spent is long.*
> *—Leonardo da Vinci*

Regardless of your age or the physical characteristics you were born with, this book is for you. We invite you to take a good look at yourself, listen to your feelings, and understand your options and the resources available as you learn how to take charge of your future. As you may have noticed, the title of our book purposefully suggests a double meaning. We want you to take a "good look" at what it really means to "look good." *The Good Look Book* takes a multifaceted approach to self-improvement because we believe that good looks are dependent on healthy living, keeping fit, and feeling good.

As physicians practicing cosmetic surgery and dermatology, we specialize in self-improvement. Through our professional association and friendship, we have spent many hours over the years discussing how our two medical specialties work together. We have found that to help our patients improve their appearances, we must also address their needs to be healthy and physically fit. This book came about as we recognized the need to combine medical options of cosmetic surgery and dermatology with other self-improvement information. *The Good Look Book* aims to give readers the total picture in one comprehensive guide.

To use a popular phrase, this book is about "being all you can be." We'll help you sort out personal, health, and lifestyle issues and identify medical and non-medical options that can increase the quality of your life, keep you looking your best at any stage of life, and prolong the active lifestyle you want to have for many years ahead.

This book is a call-to-action, a resource guide to develop your own self-improvement plan. We bring science, technology, and personal motivation together to help you live life to the fullest. We stress the importance of consulting your physician before beginning any diet or exercise program and seeking more than one qualified medical opinion on cosmetic surgery and dermatology.

Of course, this book cannot promise eternal youth, guarantee personal happiness, or give individual medical advice, but the information we present is based on results from many years of positive experiences with our patients and our sincere belief that if you are basically healthy and want to identify goals and take positive actions, you can unlock a positive self-improvement process that leads to looking better, feeling healthy, staying younger longer, and very importantly, feeling good about yourself all along the way.

Personal Bests

The chapters ahead focus on "being all you can be" for the right reasons — making self-improvement choices that suit your goals, lifestyle, and needs. Educating yourself is the first step. Gaining an objective view of what's possible and understanding what you can expect from any program means taking a realistic look at yourself. We stress the difference between making a self-improvement change for yourself, which is a healthy reason, and making a change in response to an external pressure, which is an unhealthy reason.

This book presents many of the healthiest choices in life. As you look through the table of contents, you may choose to read individual sections which match your top priorities first, or you may choose to read the chapters in order from beginning to end. The book is divided into two basic parts: the first half of the book describes the choices you have to help you feel good on the inside so you'll look good on the outside. The second half describes the choices you have to look good on the outside so you'll feel good on the inside. You'll see the strong connection between health, physical fitness, and an attractive appearance; together, they influence the way you feel about yourself.

A GREAT TIME TO BE ALIVE

> *Life can only be understood backward, but it must be lived forward.*
> *—Kierkegaard*

Today people have more lifestyle choices, medical and health care options, and educational opportunities than ever before. As a matter of fact, at the beginning of this decade the U.S. government formally announced its prescription for a healthier nation by challenging each of us to take responsibility for our health and lifestyle. This is an exciting challenge because in the years ahead, people are expected to live longer and will want to take advantage of an improved quality of life.

The Age Wave

Several years ago, *USA Today* declared that by July 1988, the 39–54 age group would outnumber the 18 to 34 year olds for the first time since the 1950s. In the mid-eighties, the first baby boomers — those born in the post–World War II years between 1946 and 1964 — started turning 40, at the front end of what the media have called the age wave. According to the 1991 census, there are now 31.5 million Americans over age 65, and that number is expected to grow to almost 39 million by the year 2000.

These statistics will have a tremendous impact in the years ahead as the estimated 66 million baby boomers begin to age. As these large numbers of people get older, aging will become the norm in our society. As they learn how to stay healthier longer, getting older won't be so hard to face, and the positive aspects of getting older will emerge stronger than ever.

This sign of the times confirms what psychologist Dr. Ross Goldstein, president of Summit Psychological Associates in San Francisco, refers to as "the new midlife," which reflects a changing standard for goods looks and healthful living. What people seem to admire most is the ability to live well, look good, and achieve maximum results from personal potential.

Findings indicate that people today are adapting positively to the natural aging process. We are actively involved in the world around us and have strong opinions — whether the concern is for the environment or political change; we approach problems with action and initiate new ideas and methods; we are interested in the quality of life and in managing our time; we tend to temper expectation with realism; we are not as rooted as our parents' generation; we do not like to foreclose any of our options; we are comfortable with progressive change; we are more concerned with who we are than what we do; and we understand that health and happiness stem from a combination of physical, mental, and emotional factors.

Famous Faces

Look around at the famous faces who grace the silver screen and tabloid pages. No longer is youth a prerequisite for famous women and men who set public examples for health and fitness. Recently Jane Fonda was photographed on the beach in a bikini looking very fit, and Cher and Raquel Welch display their toned physiques advertising for health clubs. All have figures that look just as "in shape" as any twenty year old. Although Linda Evans has matured, she's considered an example of a very "sexy, good looking woman," as is Angie Dickinson who was born in 1931, but who looks so good today that she appears in a series of advertisements with captions that read, "Would this body lie to you?"

Barbara Eden, who played the genie in "I Dream of Jeannie" on television decades ago, has popped out of her bottle once again with a nineties version of the show. Today — in her fifties — she wears the same harem pants and bares her midriff, looking incredibly like she did in the same role many years ago.

And don't forget the men! Robert Redford's rugged outdoor good looks may have aged, but he's still considered the classically handsome, all-American man. Today Steve Reeves, who was well known for his 1950s movie portrayal of Hercules, exemplifies the benefits of lifelong exercise and developed an exercise program called "power walk" which has maintained his own powerful, well-toned physique. Even the country's under-twenty set clamors for the music of the original Rolling Stones and the Grateful Dead, all of whom are men over forty.

It is impossible to think of well-known people who have been blessed with longevity and happiness without mentioning George Burns. After nearly a century of life, he maintains a positive attitude, active schedule, and youthful point of view.

Further evidence that age is just a number is found in changing marriage trends. There is a growing trend of "older" women marrying "younger" men. According to media reports, these couples marry for very solid reasons, and a large number of these marriages work out very well.

Stereotypes and myths of aging are vanishing. The pressure to "act your age" or fit a mold which suits a specific image or stage in life is gone. This kind of social progress may be the best news of all.

Fortysomething and Fiftysomething

As more people are reaching midlife in the 1990s, all indications support the prediction that you can expect to live longer than any previous generation.

Thirty-five no longer marks the beginning of mid-life. Thirty is what forty used to be, fifty is what forty used to be, and sixty is simply the beginning of the second stage of life.

But while living longer sounds great, it is important to understand that it is only an advantage if people are dedicated to insuring the quality of their lives. Fortunately, modern culture is very tuned into fitness, healthy lifestyle, wellness, preventive medicine, nutrition, and mental health — all of which make positive contributions to quality living. The choices and options are at your disposal.

Today, you can learn from the past, maximize the present, and carefully plan for the future. We are learning to be good to ourselves, and we are giving ourselves permission to be the best we can be. We're realizing that you don't have to be a movie star or television personality in order to take advantage of scientific and medical advances which can improve the quality of life and counteract the effects of time.

The Challenge of Aging

Those who have passed forty are aware of the challenge of aging. Getting back into shape or losing weight is a little tougher than it used to be. We see the fine lines and wrinkles that have begun to show at the corners of our eyes and around our mouths, and we know what it's like to lose muscle tone and store fat in unwanted places.

We all know that the natural aging process imposes limits and creates its own set of physical changes. The best athlete who reaches forty has to work even harder to maintain strength, endurance, and skill — and even with hard work cannot usually compete equally against a counterpart twenty years younger. (It *is* possible, though; veteran athletes Jimmy Connors and Nolan Ryan, among others, amazingly have sustained their tennis and baseball careers long after most players bow to the younger ones.) But today, we can do something about maintaining our looks, staying in shape, and increasing longevity. Youthful magic, natural beauty, or athletic prowess are not required. Prolonging the prime of life means treating both the body and the mind because, as the ancient Greeks knew, the mind and body are inextricably linked.

The medical part of any self-improvement process is dependent on the patient-doctor relationship. The individual who wants to improve his or her health and appearance must take an active role in the process, and both patient and doctor must communicate about realistic expectations and results.

Age and Heredity

Of course, each person has to be realistic. What you inherit from your ancestors helps determine how you look and how long you will live. Everyone knows people who live long, healthy lives in spite of unhealthy habits. You may look younger than your friends who exercise and watch what they eat, or maybe you look and feel older than people your same age.

But age and heredity will not always have the last word. While we know people who reflect exactly what their genes gave them, we know others who are, say, very physically attractive but whose parents and grandparents were not. Each of us is a product not only of genes but of lifestyle and attitude as well. You can control certain factors and make certain changes in order to maximize and maintain overall health and an attractive appearance.

Consider a few more specific examples. Loss of strength and decreasing muscle size are distinct signs of the aging process at work. However, today we know that certain kinds of exercise can counteract these problems. The body's largest organ, skin, mirrors the aging process, but there are many ways to enhance and maintain the quality of skin and skin tone. Blood pressure and percentage of body fat tend to increase with age, but they can be controlled with diet and exercise. Aging may be as plain as the nose on your face which seems to get larger as the years go by. No, it's not your imagination; the nose never stops growing, but it can be recontoured with cosmetic surgery.

The next chapter focuses on understanding yourself and creating a personal profile. Defining your self-image and identifying changes you want to make will start you on the self-improvement process. The personal information you identify in the next chapter can be used as a foundation from which to build your own action plan.

Throughout this book you will meet a few people whose outlooks have changed for the better because of the decisions they made and the actions they took to enhance their lives. Telling their own stories, they reveal genuine feelings about why they wanted to make positive changes, what it was like to do so, and how the steps they took and the results they got influenced their opinion of themselves and how others saw them.

Up Close and Personal

Will you still need me? Will you still feed me when I'm sixty-four?
                    —*The Beatles, 1967*

When you stand close to the mirror, you can see every pore, mole, and wrinkle. That's hard to take — whether you're 16 or 64. When you look at yourself close up, you tend to focus on the negatives, but if you look again, you can see positive attributes that reflect the good things about you. We're going to ask you to point out a lot about yourselves so that you can make the most of everything you have going for you.

Where you once ignored a feature that you perceived as a "negative," we want you to identify it as a possible "to be improved." For example, if your skin under your chin is fuller and looser than it used to be and you wish it were tauter, a section in this book will explain what is involved in making that improvement. If you recognize that you are storing weight in certain places and cutting back on calories isn't helping, then we'll tell you what some other options are. Let's say you come to terms with just how much you'd really like to smooth out the old acne scars on your face. We'll help you understand what's possible.

When doctors examine you close up, they look for vital signs which indicate your physical wellbeing: pulse, body temperature, blood pressure, and respiration. When your vital signs are normal, they indicate general good health, but managing long-term health and insuring the quality of life depends on evaluating many individual conditions, avoiding harmful influences, and maximizing positive influences and resources.

This chapter provides an opportunity for you to take your vital signs from head to toe — to bring out the best in you and determine the changes you want to make. You'll come to terms with what you like about yourself and determine a personal action that helps you decide what you want to improve.

Keep in mind that almost everyone has something he or she would like to improve or change. From the heavy-set woman who used to be trimmer and shapelier . . . to the man with thinning hair, baggy eyelids, and wrinkles . . . to the woman who is uncomfortable with her heavy hips and thighs . . . to the man with a large nose and receding chin . . . to the woman who tires easily and is out of shape — everyone has the potential and opportunity to change for the better. To want to improve is normal and healthy; it is not frivolous or vain.

Looking and feeling your best can increase longevity and happiness.

A recent study conducted at Rutgers University substantiates a fact that you may have suspected all along: a positive frame of mind can actually help keep you physically healthy. According to researcher Ellen Idler, who directed the study, mental outlook can influence how long a person lives. In fact, she says, "Evidence suggests that attitude is a more accurate gauge of longevity than cancer, diabetes, high blood pressure, or heart disease." The study concluded that a woman who considers herself in good health is likely to live longer than a woman who is in similar physical shape but considers herself to be in poor health.

It stands to reason that each of us has a vested interest in self-improvement activities, but many people find that "getting started" is tough and "keeping at it" is even tougher. So let's begin by eliminating the pressures that get in the way. Making positive changes need not be viewed as too difficult, too time consuming, vain, or selfish. You only need to identify your goals, decide how you're going to achieve them, and set your pace.

Attitude is key to achieving self-improvement.

Studies show that attitude affects us the same way regardless of age. If you study a group of people between the ages of thirty and seventy who are not suffering from any real diseases, you will probably find that the "unhappiest" people in the group are those who worry and suffer stress. The happiest ones, in contrast, are active and relaxed. So it is safe to say that your attitude toward life plays a big role in overall wellness. If you lighten up and give yourself room to improve, you can even get healthier. Seeking to be your best does not involve selfishness, obsessive compulsive dedication, or unrealistic thinking that you will look and feel young forever. The bottom line is if there is something about your face, your body, or your lifestyle that you do not like and wish you could change, find out if you can make a change, understand what's involved, and have an open mind about achieving that change. There are many solid reasons — both professional and personal — to want to look and feel your best at every stage of your life.

Your self-image affects your life and the lives of those around you.

Are you aware that your self-image begins to form as early as childhood? Long before it mattered to you how you looked, someone was telling you about yourself. "Oh, what a beautiful baby!" "You look just like your daddy." "She's cute but not as pretty as her sister." "Oh, what a chubby little boy!" These are the remarks that constitute the feedback we give ourselves, and they have a major influence on the opinions we form of ourselves. What we hear others say about us and the feedback we get from them sticks with us and becomes the basis for ingrained attitudes we have toward ourselves. Typically, what others say about us influences our self-concept as well as the internal dialogue, or self-talk, in which we engage. These opinions and concepts — often erroneously concocted — affect our lives in many ways, and not always for the best. Research shows, in fact, that most self-talk is negative and a conduit for anxiety and self-doubt.

By adolescence, most of us are walking around with a fairly well developed self-concept as well as a series of hang-ups about our bodies, faces, and abilities. These concepts are very influential and very resistant to change. They also affect the way we see and treat other people.

For example, fitness studies show that obese people have fewer social opportunities and make fewer career advances than those who are trim. People who exercise regularly and maintain normal weight, on the other hand, have more energy and are generally healthier than those who lead sedentary lives or are overweight. We often hear about cases where employees claim discrimination, citing incidences where an older person has been passed over or forced out in preference to a younger and more youthful-appearing person.

We know of people who spend their lives harboring inferior feelings because of poor self-concepts. We know other people who seem to "float happily through life" because they like themselves and are accepted by their peers.

In our medical practices where we specialize in helping patients look and feel their best, we constantly hear people say that they have wanted to make certain changes for a very long time. Finally, years later when they decide to go ahead and make changes, they are very happy and only wish they had done so years sooner. We find that many people grow up unconsciously adapting their personalities to fit their appearances, when in reality it would be better to adapt appearances to meet expectations. We find over and over again that patients feel better about themselves when they look the way they want to look. Many patients tell us that we have helped to bring the image they have of themselves into alignment with what they see in the mirror or in a photograph. Patients also tell us that getting involved in self-improvement and making positive changes is an inspiring and motivating personal experience.

To illustrate how people think and feel about self-improvement, we want you to read about some real people we've met in our practices. Real stories are always better than any description.

Laura (Age 42)

I had my first child in the spring when I was 32 years old. I gained a lot of weight during what I referred to as "the long winter of my pregnancy." Even though I had never had a real weight problem before, I was faced with losing about 25 pounds after delivery. This particular time in my life seemed to be a real point of reckoning. For the first time, I was overweight and definitely out of shape. I had always had a reasonable figure and had never had to really work out or diet to maintain it. My former size 7 had risen to a size 11 right after the birth of my son. Needing to lose this weight required me to face reality. Did I want go the route of many women I had seen before and let myself slip into what I considered physical mediocrity after childbirth? Or would I get busy and figure out how to reclaim my body once again?

For me, it was an easy decision, but one which certainly required a commitment. I didn't know much about weight loss and did not like to exercise unless I was actually playing a sport like tennis, but I knew I didn't want to start a physical decline in my thirties. I went to the book store, bought a book about healthy weight loss, and joined an exercise class. Within several months and in time for bathing suit weather, I was in shape and had lost the excess weight. I was proud and relieved because I'd heard a lot of people say things like, "Once you've had a baby, your body's just never the same." Well, that's not true because during this process and for the first time in my life, I began practicing healthy eating habits and regular exercise combined with a weight-training program to tone muscles. The result was the only proof I needed. My body

looked better when my son was a year old than it did before I got pregnant.

Today at age 42, I still look better than I did before I had my baby, and I continue to be challenged by the results I've achieved. This experience has also led me to take several self-improvement steps including getting involved in a good skin-care regimen, staying out of the sun, and stopping smoking. I had nasal surgery to improve my nose, and my doctor and I are working on clearing up the last of my adult acne and smoothing out the old acne scars I've had since my teenage years. The most interesting part of this story is that today I'm not bothered about aging because at a critical junction in my life, I made a decision and a commitment to be my best for the rest of my life.

Brad (Age 35)

I was very secure about my physical build when I was in high school and college because I was lucky to be born with height, strong shoulders, and a slim waist, but I always felt that my face just didn't match my body. They just didn't go together. I had this strong, masculine body — which I worked to develop — but my face really fell short of what I wished it could be. I felt that my only choice was to accept what I had. I certainly didn't want to be a Michael Jackson and change my appearance and become unrecognizable. I just wanted certain features to be slightly different, but I never really considered the possibilities of cosmetic surgery until I had a sports injury and my nose was broken.

When I saw a plastic surgeon, we discussed my nose and what could be done to treat the injury. The next thing I knew I was telling him how I felt about my face. To make a long story short, the doctor reshaped my nose, made it slightly smaller, and improved my jawline and chin contour. My face is more masculine, and I definitely think I look much better. The result has made a big difference for me. Even though the physical change is subtle, I really see myself in a very different light, and I am extremely motivated and much more self-confident. My face matches my body. Now they look like they go together. It's like meeting someone whose personality matches his appearance. It makes sense to me because I've spent years wanting to look the way I do today. I couldn't be happier about taking this action or about the results.

Sarah (Age 52)

My husband and I got a divorce two years ago after 26 years of marriage and three grown children. I felt lost and at first, a little panicked at the thought of being alone. I felt really gloomy about my prospects when I started realizing that, in order to meet new people, I'd have to face the world and play the game after all these years. This was the hardest time in my entire life, and for awhile I was very depressed and very resentful.

I finally decided that I had to do something to make myself feel better because I didn't want to live the rest of my life this way. It was hard though because I felt very demobilized. I joined a singles' group consisting of men and women in my same situation. The group offered a lot of activities — one of which was biking for beginners. I held my breath and signed up — even though I had not ridden a bicycle since I was a child. I went twice a week for practice and took the day trip on Saturdays. This may sound crazy, but I felt more exhilarated than I had in years. Just being active and feeling athletic again made me a new person and helped me see the world in a different perspective. I was meeting people and had something new to look forward to.

That year, I went back to work which helped me make more new friends. I lost 15 pounds, had a facelift, and had my eyelids done. The biking really improved my muscle tone and my figure. My children say I've never looked better. I'm dating someone very special now, and life looks pretty great. It takes a while sometimes to turn your life around, but it can be done. As a matter of fact, my life is better now than it has been in many years. I'm certainly much happier and feel and look better than I have in a long time.

These personal accounts are representative of the kinds of stories we hear in our medical practices. Too often it takes an event, such as an injury in the case of Brad, or a passage in life, such as childbirth for Laura or divorce for Sarah, to bring a person to the point where he or she feels the need to change something or initiate self-improvement. However, it isn't necessary for an event or passage in life to occur before you take action. What we hear over and over again from our patients is, "I just wish I'd done this years ago." Perhaps the greatest reward of all our self-improvement efforts is that we bring the best out in ourselves, and we take advantage of our potential — not only for a healthier body and an improved appearance but for a happier, more rewarding life.

In actuality, self-improvement is about getting off the couch, out from behind the desk, away from the same old routine and bursting through stereotypes, hang-ups, self-talk, insecurities, and fears. You don't have to compete with anyone, measure yourself by other people's standards, or aspire toward any set image. Self-improvement is the very best way to prove something wonderful to yourself.

The Beauty Myth

It is very important to remember that we stress a multifaceted, interdependent approach to self-improvement. For too long our society has perpetuated the myth that mere physical appearance is the standard of beauty without considering all the components of a genuinely attractive, healthy, happy person.

Such stereotypical thinking stymies both men and women and ignores the changing roles they face today. Naomi Wolf, author of the best-selling book *The Beauty Myth*, deals with the stereotypical image of beauty and its effect on women. Ms. Wolf makes a strong case for ways in which "the beauty myth" has hindered the advancement of older women. She points out that many times older women are passed over or even let go from a job and replaced by a younger, more attractive woman who has less professional experience and personal knowledge of the job.

In our practices and experiences with patients, we have seen how the perpetuation of a beauty myth has influenced and even hindered the advancement of older women, but the effect of a beauty myth has not stopped there. It affects women of all ages, and it affects men too.

The media's frequent equation of youth and beauty and the pressure imposed by a culture heretofore obsessed with youthful images have molded and shaped the lives of many people of all ages. So many carve their personal appearance goals and physical aspirations from a stereotyped standard set by the media, the fashion industry, or the movies. When this happens, the expectations are as unrealistic as the standard itself.

Many think this is primarily a women's issue perpetuated by a male-dominated society, but it is interesting to note that men quite often feel they too have been adversely affected by a male equivalent of a stereotypical appearance standard that exists in our society today. More and more, we hear men patients say that they are being judged by unrealistic standards, and that they feel threatened by the younger man on the job or have lost a girlfriend or wife to a younger and more attractive man. These men come to us because they seek a competitive edge and a way to feel better about who they are and how they look — just as women come to us for the same reasons.

The answer, of course, is to rid ourselves of myths about how we should look and stop responding to external pressures. We can stop imposing the myths on others by not incorporating them into our own judgment and rededicate ourselves to a creative, individual standard that is directed toward making the most of each individual at each stage of his or her life. This is a people issue and one that affects both males and females from youth to maturity.

What we have come to understand is that although many factors in our society are not equal, most of the people we see respond equally to pressures associated with individual success in this highly competitive world. While the majority of our patients are women, the men who come to see us share some of the same concerns.

Certainly, men and women face competition from those who are younger and possibly more attractive. But an increasing number of them admit that although a youthful appearance plays a role in professional and personal advancement, it is not the ultimate deciding factor. Experience, judgment, and expertise are major factors in the modern workplace.

We see fewer and fewer women patients who seek cosmetic procedures (either surgical or nonsurgical) which will create changes linked to a stereotypical image of beauty. More women say, for example, "I want to improve the proportions of my body," rather than "I want to look like this picture." And there is a difference. The first statement reflects the woman's desire to improve herself. She is relating to her features and wanting to put them in proportion to her body. The second statement indicates that the woman is not so much in touch with her own features as she is trying to mold them to fit a stereotypical image of a picture she admires.

Our experience shows that both women and men want to be their best, but they are increasingly aware of their own self-images and do not compare themselves to others. This is still a tough job, as people today continue to be bombarded with commercial advertisements and slick messages which attempt to perpetuate "the beauty myth."

Working with many different kinds of women and men of all ages, we see times and attitudes are changing. There is much more concern with the individual components of an attractive, healthy person. These components include good health, physical fitness, emotional and mental health, a positive attitude, and a value for personal and professional experience. We see that more people feel secure about projecting their own styles which stem not from fashion but from their professional and personal interests. We see increased initiative, creativity, and motivation.

The bottom line is that being your best and making the most of yourself will probably always be an individual advantage; people who are concerned with making positive changes in order to improve or maintain an attractive appearance and a balanced, healthy approach to life and longevity are generally more desirable, happier, secure, and successful than those who are not. Today, more people are aware of the fact that being thin does not mean you are physically fit. A pretty or handsome face does not connote health. Just because you are attractive or young does not mean you are happy or that you feel good about yourself. We see many "beautiful" people who are unsuccessful, unhappy, and physically unfit. Yet we see increasing numbers of people — especially growing numbers of professionally successful women and men — whose values include a mixture of experience, talent, good looks, and good health.

As a person matures, it is very important to focus on what can be done to counteract the natural aging process such as a loss of muscle mass or the disappearance of smooth skin, but it is just as important to focus on the many ways in which maturity brings rewards and gains.

As author Naomi Wolf points out, "Older women are more energetic, more powerful, and more comfortable with their abilities." This description certainly holds true of the older women we now see in our medical practices, but women of all ages are taking more risks and headed in new directions. It seems that Madison Avenue and Hollywood are beginning to take the lead from these women rather than the other way around. We see evidence that indicates stereotypes are increasingly unpopular, and individuals are growing increasingly secure within themselves. Being the best you can be — throughout all the passages of life — is the key to success.

Since modern medicine and science have progressed beyond areas of critical response, women and men of all ages can elect to change and grow. It is now well within the practical realm of possibility for almost any person to embark on a self-improvement program. No need to put off until tomorrow what will make you better today. The first step is relatively simple. Just take a close look at yourself in a very objective and sensitive manner.

Mirror, Mirror on the Wall

In preparation for the self-check exercises which follow on the next few pages, let's do a little head work. Remember, you're doing these exercises for yourself, and the more objective you can be, the better your results. Don't be timid about identifying areas of your face or body that you'd like to change because in most cases, there's a formula for improving "that something" you don't like.

All of us look into two different mirrors: the glass mirror that reflects our image and the mirror in our minds which reflects our self-image. No matter how you actually look to others, the image you have of yourself is the stronger of the two. This self-image is the result of years of conditioning and self-talk that occurs when you form opinions about what you think you look like in the mirror or in photographs. The emphasis is on what you tell yourself. And, technically speaking, a mirror image is not as telling as a photograph. Unretouched photographs tend to give a more realistic image of how you really look. A mirror image is actually a reversed image and one that you're so accustomed to seeing that it may have lost its impact. Although you'll be asked to use the mirror as you answer the questions on the next few pages, be sure you keep in mind how you look in photos — and, most importantly, what you're thinking and saying to yourself.

As you work through the instructions and questions, simply think about the answers. You don't need to write down anything yet; just take some quiet time and listen to yourself. Don't get overwhelmed. This is your chance — in the privacy of your own home — to take an uncensored view of yourself.

1. For starters, close your eyes and picture yourself. What do you see? What are your strengths as a person? What do you like about yourself? What do others like about you?

2. Next, stand in front of the mirror and stare very carefully at your freshly washed face and neck (without makeup). Study yourself from the front, side, and three-quarter views. Look at your forehead, hairline, your eyes, nose, and mouth. What do you see? What do you like about your face? What do you dislike? Do you notice any recent changes in your facial contours? Do you have wrinkles or lines that bother you? Do you have heavy folds in the skin around your mouth? Do you have baggy, saggy eyelids that don't go away when you're rested? Do you have any scars that bother you? Do you have sun damage? Does the skin on your neck sag or do you have a double chin? Does your skin look and feel soft and supple? Do you look tired? Is your hair thinning or are you balding? What is your best feature? What do people usually comment about when they compliment you?

3. Still standing in front of the mirror, study your physique from the front, side, and three-quarter views. You should do this both dressed and undressed because clothes can emphasize or deemphasize certain areas and enhance or mask the physique you see in a bathing suit or when you are undressed.

The first question is, do you like what you see? How's your weight? Are you overweight or underweight? Are you storing excess fat in specific areas? Even with exercise and proper diet, are there problem areas which you cannot control? Do you have good muscle tone? Can you see muscular definition in your body? Is your skin soft and supple? Do you have sun damaged skin? Do you have any cellulite, excess fat in the breast or chest area, flabby upper arms or legs, love handles, or saddlebags? What are your best features? What part or parts of your body do you emphasize? What part or parts of your body do you de-emphasize?

4. Now, go to the family album and take a nice, leisurely visual stroll down memory lane. Look at your photographs — from childhood through adolescence to the present. What do you see? How have you changed over the years? What features have remained constant?

What family characteristics do you notice that you share with relatives? For example, perhaps you notice that your skin — like your sibling's — was smooth and clear until about age 15. Then you broke out with acne. The acne has gone away, but the scars haven't, and you've forgotten how you looked with smooth skin. You also notice that although the women in your family tend to age gracefully, they are prone to carry extra weight in the hips and buttocks. Most of them started putting on pounds after age forty, but your mother gained her weight steadily with the birth of each child and never lost it.

Do you also notice that in many of your photos — from early teenage years on — that there are any particular features which have consistently bothered you throughout the years? Say it's your nose which is a little bit crooked or too prominent. As a matter of fact, do you notice that your nose, which you inherited from your father, looks great on him, but is really too large for your smaller face? Or can you see how much younger you looked with a different hair style, less weight, or more hair?

As you consider your facial and body characteristics, keep in mind that you are born with certain inherited features and pre-determined characteristics. You have no control over what you inherit from previous generations of family members. Facial features and body structures, as well as longevity and even the process of how you age, are determined by genetics, but remember that you can make a big difference in what you inherited — in health, longevity, and physical attractiveness. Being your best depends on your attitude and the commitment you make to the quality of your present and future life.

How Do You Handle Change?

How flexible are you when it comes to making changes? You are probably reading this book because you are either gathering information about change or you are considering making a change, but how willing are you to make the commitment?

Let's examine some basic elements surrounding people's desire to change. Research shows that people change because they are tired of hurting or have hit rock bottom, because they are bored and decide to try something new, or — very importantly — because they suddenly discover that change is a new option for them. For most people, the knowledge that change is possible produces excitement about new opportunities. The knowledge that it's okay to change is liberating, and exposure to others who have experienced change increases the individual possibilities for change.

As physicians, we also see some negative thinkers who are dissatisfied, unhappy, or unhealthy but do not want to change. Perhaps you know people who fit this description. Theoretically, many of these people are actually dependent on complaining or feeling sorry for themselves. As the Carly Simon song goes, "Suffering was the only way I knew I was alive." If a dissatisfied, unhappy, or unhealthy person makes a potentially positive change, they will no longer have their "problems" to cling to. Getting well and becoming happier and healthier threatens what they are accustomed to.

If these negative thinkers were to change for the better, they would have to give up their comfortable old habits. They would lose the security blankets they use to get attention and sympathy from family, friends, and co-workers. After all, it is hard to feel sorry for a

healthy, happy, attractive person. To negative thinkers, the thought of changing for the better is rather threatening because they do not know how to relate to others and feel uncomfortable interacting as healthy, happy, attractive people. Subconsciously, if not consciously, although these people are accustomed to dealing with misery and suffering, they experience little joy, positive fulfillment, and self-confidence.

Unfortunately, pain or unhappiness can control your life, but these situations are treatable, and healing can occur if the individual acknowledges the problem and seeks help and support. However, in some cases, even though help is available, the individual resists taking the necessary steps to change.

On the other hand, most of us fall into the category of very normal people who would like to improve something about ourselves but either have a hard time getting started or cling to our habits more easily than embarking on new ones. It is comfortable to stay the way you are and challenging to make a change. We are creatures of habit, and old habits die hard.

So, if you find that you'd like to make a change, but you feel stuck when it comes to getting started, the first rule of thumb is to understand that maintaining flexibility and keeping an open mind are important parts of your positive decision-making process. In simple terms, when you try a new way of doing things — whether it's eating different foods, changing the way you use your time throughout the day, or actively deciding to change the way you look and feel about yourself, you will have new experiences which will expand your perspective. Therefore, the ability to change can be a very positive process, but you won't know just how positive it can be until you make a commitment to change.

These are the key points to focus on when dealing with change:

• Remember that change is possible and that it is okay to change.

• If you want to change something about yourself or modify your behavior, identify the change you want to make and learn everything you can about the opportunities and facts associated with that change. Gather information, talk to experts, and interview others who have had experience making a similar change. Make sure you objectively understand any risks associated with the change you are considering.

• In order to make a successful change, it is necessary to incorporate your mind — as well as your body — in the process. How you think, what you tell yourself, and how you behave will affect results either positively or negatively. Even the most successful changes do not guarantee personal happiness. That part is up to each individual.

• Making changes involving health — such as improving eating habits or increasing physical activity patterns — should be approached methodically and started gradually. Successful change is not a "quick fix." It is always recom-

mended that you consult your doctor before making dietary changes or beginning exercise programs.

• Making physical changes involving dermatology and cosmetic surgery have enhanced many lives and improved many appearances, but they do not perform miracles. The realistic and objective results which dermatology and plastic surgery provide offer improvement — not perfection.

• Making positive changes involves education and commitment. Properly managed, this process can be very rewarding and gratifying.

• Changes can occur slowly and gradually with some progress being made on a regular basis. Take things one step at a time. You can take "baby steps" much easier than you can take "giant steps." If you want to make a change, make up your mind to do so and then just focus on making some progress every day. Days turn into weeks, and weeks into months, and months into . . . history.

As we begin the important self-analysis process, let's take a careful look at the person we see when we look in the mirror or in photographs. In the next several sections, you will be able to identify areas of your face and body as well as personal health and lifestyle issues which you might like to change or improve. Don't get overwhelmed. There's no one who wouldn't like to change something about themselves.

The idea behind these exercises is simply to identify any feature or condition which could be improved and match your list of check marks to the various sections of this book which outline specific self-improvement options. By matching your goals with the information about health, fitness, nutrition, and medical self-improvement options throughout this book, you will emerge with an action plan for the future.

Facescape

Review your thoughts from the analysis over the previous pages. Let's begin with your face — the part most people see first. Are there any facial or neck areas which could be improved? In the space provided, check those areas that you'd like to improve.

_____ sagging neck skin
_____ drooping or double chin
_____ weak or receding chin
_____ protruding chin
_____ cheek jowls
_____ down-turned corners of the mouth
_____ thin or fat lips
_____ creases or folds between the nose and corners of the mouth
_____ flat or weak cheeks
_____ large nose
_____ wide, flared nostrils
_____ crooked or humped nose

_____ protruding or prominent ears
_____ enlarged skin pores
_____ fine lines around the eyes
_____ dark circles or puffiness under the eyes
_____ puffiness or droopiness of upper eyelids or brows
_____ crow's feet at corners of the eyes
_____ fine lines above and below the lips
_____ furrows and deep lines on the forehead
_____ hair thinning or loss
_____ facial scarring caused by acne
_____ facial scarring caused by injury or illness
_____ uneven texture of facial skin
_____ acne and blemishes
_____ dry, peeling skin
_____ oily skin
_____ overall tired, haggard look
_____ relaxed facial muscles
_____ excess facial fat
_____ spider-web blood vessels
_____ sun-damaged skin (excess freckles, pigmentation, keratosis)
_____ skin rash or irritation
_____ unsightly moles, birthmarks, growths, age spots
_____ other (describe)

_____
_____
_____
_____
_____
_____

Next, review the items you checked and prioritize them. List the items in order of what concerns you most.

1._____ 7._____

2._____ 8._____

3._____ 9._____

4._____ 10._____

5._____ 11._____

6._____ 12._____

Body Mapping

Now, let's move to the rest of your body. Map out the problem areas by checking the ones that you'd like to improve.

_____sun damage to upper chest skin
_____sagging skin at the upper arms
_____concerns with breasts (women)
  _____too large
  _____too small
  _____asymmetrical
  _____drooping
  _____changes after childbirth and nursing
_____concerns with chest (men)
  _____flabby skin caused by weight gain and loss
  _____excessive fatty tissue caused by discontinued weight training
  _____excessive skin and fatty areas at abdomen
_____excessive skin and fatty areas at midriff
_____weak abdominal muscles
_____excessive fatty deposits at the hips

_____excessive fatty thighs
_____excessive fatty buttocks
_____excessive fatty knees
_____excessive fatty calves
_____excessive fatty ankles
_____cellulite
  _____arms
  _____thighs
  _____buttocks
  _____abdomen area
_____varicose veins or broken capillaries on legs or thighs
_____body scarring
_____unusual changes in the skin such as raised, dark, scaly, irritated, or bleeding spots
_____moles or birthmarks
_____age spots on hands or other areas
_____general lack of muscle tone
_____overall sagging quality of skin
_____overall wrinkled quality of skin
_____stretch marks
_____other (describe)

_____

_____

_____

Now, review the areas you checked and prioritize them. List them in the order of which ones concern you most.

1._____ 7._____

2._____ 8._____

3._____ 9._____

4._____ 10._____

5._____ 11._____

6._____ 12._____

The next exercise relates to lifestyle and routine habits. Respond based on your lifestyle as it is today, not on any start-stop programs you have previously experienced. The idea here is to identify the habits and physical conditions which can harm your health. For example, if you smoke or if your percentage of body fat is high, the information in this book may help to convince you to give up cigarettes or tell you how to lower your amount of body fat.

By matching your goals with the information about health, fitness, nutrition, and medical self-improvement options throughout this book, you will emerge with direction for the future.

Health Habits

Answer *yes* or *no* to each lifestyle question or statement below.

_____I smoke less than one pack per day.
_____I smoke one pack per day.
_____I smoke more than one pack per day.
_____I smoke a pipe or cigar.
_____I use chewing tobacco.
_____I like to drink and consume 1–2 drinks per day.
_____I like to drink and consume 3 or more drinks per day.
_____Sometimes I drink too much and feel bad the next day.
_____Alcoholism runs in my family.

Personal Profile

My blood pressure is:

_____Below 121/71
_____121/71 to 140/85
_____141/86 to 170/100
_____171/101 to 190/110
_____Above 191/111

My blood cholesterol level is:

_____150 or below
_____150 to 200
_____201 to 239
_____240 to 300
_____over 300

My HDL cholesterol level is:

_____over 60
_____60 to 45
_____44 to 36
_____35 to 28
_____27 to 22

My weight is:

_____Normal
_____10% above normal
_____Overweight (approximately 15–30 percent)
_____Overweight (more than 30 percent)
_____Percentage of body fat is between 10 and 20 percent
_____Percentage of body fat is between 21 and 30 percent
_____Percentage of body fat is over 30 percent

Personality and Stress

_____Uncomfortable discussing personal problems and feelings
_____Very competitive
_____Feel angry and hostile
_____Depressed
_____Overworked with little social or leisure activity
_____Always striving to please others

_____Accident prone
_____Lose my temper easily
_____Suffer from headaches, dizziness,
nervous stomach, back pain, or
heart palpitations

Exercise Habits

_____I rarely exercise.
_____I exercise sometimes —
approximately 2 times weekly.
_____I exercise 30 – 45 minutes three
times weekly.
_____I exercise at least 45 minutes four
to five times weekly.
_____I exercise every day for at least
30 – 45 minutes.
_____My routine includes 30 – 45
minutes of cardiovascular exercise.
_____My exercise routine involves
weight-resistance activity.
_____My exercise program involves
cross-training activities.

Fitness Level

_____I am very physically fit.
_____My fitness level is above average.
_____My fitness level is average.
_____My fitness level is below average.
_____My fitness level is very low.

Diet Habits

_____I eat a lot of rich dairy products
such as butter, cream, and cheese.
_____I eat meats frequently.
_____I like to salt my food.
_____I eat more than three eggs per
week.
_____I eat rich desserts such as ice
cream and cakes frequently.
_____I eat lowfat or nonfat dairy

products (milk, cheese, yogurt,
2 – 3 servings per day).
_____I eat foods that are high in fiber
(bran cereals, wheat breads, brown
rice; 6 – 8 servings per day).
_____I eat vegetables daily (3 – 4
servings per day).
_____I eat fruits daily (2 – 3 servings).
_____I eat protein from lowfat or lean
sources (poultry, fish, lean meat,
beans; 4 – 7 ounces per day).
_____I fast to lose weight.
_____I use fad diets to lose weight.
_____I drink 6 – 8 glasses of water daily.
_____I am a late diner or eat late-night
snacks.
_____I eat breakfast.
_____I eat small portions regularly,
several times per day.
_____I take dietary supplements based
on my body's requirements.

In the spaces below, write — in
order of your priority — the lifestyle
issues and health habits which fall into
the "to be improved" category. As you
read through the various sections of the
book, you can match your priorities to
the options and solutions which are
available.

1. _____
2. _____
3. _____
4. _____
5. _____
6. _____
7. _____
8. _____
9. _____
10. _____
11. _____
12. _____

SECRETS OF EATING SMART

No way around it . . .
you are what you eat.

A moderate program of healthy eating and physical activity can actually increase your body's ability to slow down the aging process — no matter what your age. This simply confirms the fact that each individual can improve on heredity factors and prolong the prime of life.

There is no standard that marks a person as being *past prime*. People age according to individual patterns which are based on varying factors — some we can control, others we cannot. Obviously, slowing down the aging process means increasing the body's abilities to prolong health.

Over the years, the body reduces its total number of healthy cells. In the aging process, the body gradually loses its reserves and eventually loses its ability to regenerate them. This gradual loss is due, in large part, to the decreasing number of cells in each organ of the body.

The secretion of the growth hormone also diminishes with age. In addition to regulating growth, the growth hormone stimulates the immune system and influences the body's ability to repair itself. Plus, as aging occurs, the body tends to lose muscle mass and bone density as well as strength, vitality, and skin tone. With age, the body also tends to increase the amount of fat it keeps as energy storage tissue — even if the overall size and weight of the body has not increased significantly. This extra body fat is typically stored in specific locations around the body, some of which signal risk factors such as heart disease, stroke, and diabetes.

When the body increases its ability to slow down the aging process through a combination of such factors as nutrition and exercise, it becomes stabilized. In some cases, a reversal of the aging process occurs, improving the body's ability to store resources, build up resistance, and guard against deterioration.

There are many different benefits associated with slowing down the aging process. Scientific evidence suggests we can actually reduce the onset of debilitating conditions and diseases such as senility, cataracts, arthritis, diabetes, and loss of sexual fulfillment. Optimally, prolonging the prime of life means adding years to the midlife — not extending the years referred to as "old age."

23

The First Step

Slowing down the aging process begins with nutrition. Yet curiously, many people have not taken steps toward "eating smart."

A recent survey conducted for the American Dietetic Association showed that while 79 percent of the people questioned think nutrition is important, only 44 percent believe they are doing all they can to eat a healthy diet. The reasons for not eating smart varied among respondents, but 38 percent cited an unwillingness to give up favorite foods and 25 percent said that keeping track of what they ate was too much trouble. These are pale excuses when you consider the facts.

The problem may be that many people are responding to confusion and fear over what and how much to eat. So many of our patients say they are "afraid" they are eating too much fat, too much cholesterol, and getting too many hidden chemicals in their diets, but they admit they "aren't sure just how to get good nutrition." It seems that we are overwhelmed by media reports about foods, food additives, food preparation, pesticides, and fertilizers. As a result, many people feel guilty and bad about eating, and this is definitely not healthy. Others respond by saying, "Oh, well, until they find out what the truth really is, I'm just going to eat whatever I please."

Neither situation is acceptable. The answer lies in the word *balance*. Food is meant to be enjoyed. The phenomenon of eating disorders such as anorexia is an increasing modern problem that is born out of negative feelings associated with food and its effect on the body. The most healthy, nutritious diet is a balance of many foods. The concern is not for certain "good" or "bad" foods. The concern is for a balanced combination of foods.

FACT: The quality of what goes into the body determines, to a great extent, the quality of the body's reserves and defenses. Thus eating smart is the first step toward increased longevity and better health. Did you know that each year the body replaces over 90 percent of its total atoms with new ones? These new atoms come from the food we eat, the water we drink, and the air we breathe.

FACT: Heredity is only half the story. Of course, heredity plays a major part in how healthy and resistant to disease the body is, but heredity does not control the adult decision-making process. History clearly indicates that men and women have the abilities to be better than their ancestors. Therefore, the decisions you make and the actions you take dramatically affect your longevity and health.

FACT: Education and an awareness of the facts are the necessary tools for eating smart. Like every other self-improvement step, the decision to eat smart need not be an overwhelming, drastic change. Balancing change against existing personal habits can be approached in a "one step at a time" manner. As the American Dietetic Association points out, "No one need give up their favorite foods, and even candy bars can be eaten in moderation."

FACT: Tracking every bite you eat is unnecessary. It may be effective for people on a specific diet program or for those attempting to identify their behavior patterns; but tracking your food is not necessary in order to begin eating smarter and improving nutrition habits. Every time you reach for something to eat, you are in position to make a decision about what you are going to choose to eat.

FACT: How much do you weigh? How many calories do you eat per day? Counting calories and measuring body weight are no longer the total picture. The emphasis is on matching a balance of foods to individual needs and health objectives. Counting fat, carbohydrates, and protein is as important as counting calories. Weighing in is as important as measuring percentage of body fat. How do your clothes fit? How many inches can you pinch at your midriff or on your outer thigh? If excess weight is a problem, are you eating increased amounts of complex carbohydrates such as vegetables, fruits, pasta, and whole grains instead of large portions of meat and dairy products in order to satisfy your appetite? Complex carbohydrates make the body work harder to store away fat. Are you eating smart or just eating?

FACT: Eating smart may require behavior modification, involving the mind as well as the body. Any self-improvement that comes about through changing your normal habits is generally longer lasting than dramatic changes which demand an "all at once" difference. The desire to improve your eating habits and an awareness of nutrition facts are the keys to successful, long-term results.

FACT: Since eating smarter is based on personal decisions you can control, you have a terrific opportunity to use change in a positive way. Obviously, eating smart involves choices regarding food selection, food preparation, nutrition, and weight control, but the initial concern is learning to recognize your eating patterns and discovering your vulnerabilities. Many people who make less-than-smart eating decisions do so out of ignorance about nutritional sources and their benefits to the body or in response to habit and environment rather than hunger. Smart eating applies to everyone, regardless of age, whether you are normal weight, overweight, or underweight.

FACT: Eating smart is key to weight reduction and weight control. When overweight people lose weight and maintain the loss, this change increases their sense of physical and emotional well-being and reduces the health risks associated with being overweight or obese. Excessive body weight and body fat point to increased risk of coronary artery disease, hypertension, and hypertensive heart disease, as well as diabetes, certain types of cancer (such as breast and uterine cancers in women and colon, rectal, and prostatic cancers in men), arthritis, respiratory disease, gallbladder disease, and stroke. Weight loss — even in moderate amounts — tends to reduce hypertensive blood pressure and increase life expectancy for overweight people.

FACT: Keeping yourself trim is not enough because a trim person is not necessarily a healthy person. Too many people are obsessed with "thinness"— probably because they do not really understand how the body works or how the aging process occurs, or because they are caught up with a false image of what constitutes an attractive appearance. Once you know the facts about the link between nutrition, health, and aging, it is hard to ignore the evidence and remain focused on false and incomplete standards of measurement, such as mere weight and physical size.

FACT: In cases involving obesity, getting people to modify their eating habits and manage their diets has not proven to be very successful. Track records show that the overwhelming majority relapse and regain the weight they lost. Modern research tells us that uncontrollable eating patterns are best treated as problems of addiction with emphasis put on helping these people counteract their self-defeating emotions, develop long-term behavior changes,

and get into strong support groups. Many who suffer from overeating are actually eating as a response to stress or other emotional triggers, and these responses produce irrational thinking and behavior. It is very important that these people understand the emotional side of their problem.

The Pleasure Syndrome

Do we eat and drink too much? The answer is probably *yes* because most of us live to eat rather than eat to live. We are not suggesting that food should not be enjoyed; it should indeed. But like the Romans of centuries ago, our modern society tends to be overly indulgent. In order to promote smart eating practices, it is vital to recognize why our society eats and drinks too much.

First of all, eating and drinking are major focal points of almost all social and many business activities. It is very difficult for the average person to avoid what we refer to as recreational eating and drinking. Many of us make poor eating decisions because we are constantly confronted by food and drink everywhere we go. Simply following the crowd can lead to excesses in food and alcohol — especially when a busy social calendar or business obligations are involved. This is why we refer to eating and drinking as a part of the pleasure syndrome, a term referring to any activity that makes us feel good but has little or no lasting value and which can lead to destructive habits and behavior patterns.

Eating and the Mind

Another force which has a major impact on our lifestyles and eating habits is commercial advertising. We are constantly being marketed to and persuaded to eat and drink the way other people direct us. These commercial promoters use delicious-looking powers of suggestions. We see and hear their messages on television and in magazines and newspapers. Most appetites are conditioned by the repetitive commercial presentation of food.

Increasingly, people eat in restaurants or stand in line for certain taste sensations at fast-food places. Many of us eat out regularly for convenience and end up selecting our principal diets from what is available on menus. We are conditioned to desire foods which, like "the beauty myth" mentioned in the previous chapter, may look good on the surface but are missing key ingredients. And unfortunately, a whole new generation of young people has grown up with fast foods and fatty diets during their formative years.

The aromas of foods, as well as the mental pictures we conjure up when we are hungry, trigger our appetites. The trick is to create your own set of standards for appealing foods — based on an educated approach to what the body needs in order to work well and prolong the prime of life. This is the kind of decision-making process that engages the "smart" part of the brain — the part that allows us to take control of what we are eating and drinking.

For example, have you ever questioned why they put the desserts at the front of the cafeteria line? When you're hungry, you tend to eat with your eyes. If you fill your tray with other foods, you would be less likely to buy dessert at the end of the line. They hope to trigger your appetite so that you will have dessert in addition to the other basic dishes you put on your tray. Once you begin to think about these kinds of mind games, you will be more prone to act intelligently rather than respond to impulse.

Appetite Triggers

Let's take a look at some of the ways in which both external and internal forces trigger the appetite:

- power of persuasion (visual and aromatic)
- part of socializing; peer pressure
- physical fatigue
- boredom; lack of activity
- nervousness; anxiety
- habit (versus eating only when hungry)
- need for convenience
- loneliness
- anger

- behavior rationalization
- food shopping while hungry
- lack of education
- routine schedule

There are hundreds of triggers, but these common ones are good illustrations of the forces that work on our appetites. We see many patients who successfully improve their eating habits once they understand why the body requires certain nutrients to continue working well for a long time. Awareness is the trick.

Eating Behavior

Understanding your eating behavior is important whether you would like to lose weight, want to improve nutrition, or both. Answer these questions in order to see how you eat.

Do you eat too fast?

Eating too fast means you probably finish before anyone else, put more food into your mouth before you have thoroughly swallowed the previous bite, and fail to realize you are full and keep eating. Appetite lags behind eating by 20 to 30 minutes.

Do you eat too much at one time?

Eating too much at one time means you probably feel uncomfortable after eating, do not fully taste your food, eat while you're on the run (maybe in the car or at your desk at work), and eat when you're not really hungry.

Do you eat because something triggers your appetite?

Appetite triggers, such as the ones listed just above, can be external or emotional. Even though these triggers form the basis for many poor eating habits, it is vital to understand that each person can control his or her behavior. Changing behavior — by beginning to change the decisions you make regarding your eating habits — is a very positive way to get control of what you eat, why you eat, when you eat, and how you eat. This technique involves behavior modification.

Behavior modification means making intelligent changes in the actions you decide to take until you have conditioned yourself to change your behavior. It has been said that "the problem is not the problem. The problem is my *attitude* about the problem." The human mind has tremendous capabilities for problem-solving, but most of us mere humans have a power struggle between doing what we are accustomed to and changing our behavior in order to improve ourselves and our lives.

This is the real personal point of reckoning. No doctor, friend, parent, or spouse can harness the power of your mind and strengthen your will for you.

Positive Changes Are Not Difficult

How can you combat those ever-ready appetite triggers when they seem to be controlling your behavior? Let's take a good look.

• If you are eating in response to emotional triggers such as anger or loneliness, talk about the emotions you are experiencing with someone who will be supportive and helpful. Train yourself to channel the negative energy associated with your anger, frustration, loneliness, etc., toward something you know you enjoy. Try sitting down or reclining as calmly as possible and begin to visualize a pleasant scene or happy memory.

• To relieve stress and increase your ability to relax, use these simple muscular relaxation and breathing techniques:

Breathing Technique:
Sit in a chair with both feet on the floor and both hands resting on the upper thighs. Your palms are open and facing the ceiling. Your eyes are closed. Begin to inhale by taking a very deep breath, keeping your chest still and pushing out your diaphragm (abdomen), to the count of eight — one thousand and one, one thousand and two, one thousand and three, etc. When you have reached the count of one thousand and eight, begin to exhale very slowly, again counting in the same manner to eight. Repeat this process at least 10 to 15 consecutive times, inhaling and exhaling slowly and rhythmically. You should begin to feel a definite change of mood characterized by heightened calm and relaxation.

Muscular Relaxation Technique:
Starting at your feet (or your face), select one part of the body at a time. Tense the muscles in your feet very tightly and hold that tension to the same count of eight you used in the breathing exercise. When you reach the one thousand and eight count, slowly release the tension, counting again to eight in the same manner. Move to the next part of the body — the legs — and repeat the process until you have worked your way up or down the entire body. This simple muscular exercise is great for relieving physical tensions and increasing your ability to relax. Both the muscular and the breathing exercises can help you change negative energy into positive energy because they both enhance relaxation and reduce tension, which helps you get into a better mood or frame of mind.

• If you find that you are eating because you are tired, take a relaxing bath or a refreshing shower instead. Try to lie down and rest, turning off your mind to the activities of the day and any stressful situations.

- If you are lonely, make yourself get out and go somewhere. Initiate an activity. Find a companion. Read the newspaper's calendar of events and find an adventure. Go to a movie. Make that "to do" list or tackle a chore you've been putting off. Pursue new or interesting activities.

- If you are eating as a response to a picture on television or because something smells great, immediately remove the external stimulation. Involve your mind in something else.

- If you find yourself eating unnecessarily because food and drink are all around you at social or business functions, be sure to eat very small portions and eat slowly. Don't be timid about refusing food or drink when you really do not want any. If alcohol is a problem, why not order a glass of sparkling water with a twist of lime?

- If you are eating as a response to nervous energy or because you feel depressed or anxious, force yourself to do something physical. Walk, jog, rake the lawn, sweep the floor, vacuum the carpets, or sing out loud. Also, this is a good time to apply muscular relaxation and breathing exercises.

- Last but not least, if you are rationalizing your behavior with statements such as "I can't help it," "I'll be different tomorrow," or "It doesn't matter because no one really knows what's good for you anyway," then just know deep down that you are not telling yourself the truth.

Many of our patients come to us not to study nutrition but because they are dissatisfied with some aspect of their bodies. In many cases what they want to change about themselves is directly linked to one or more of three sources: being overweight or underweight, being out-of-shape, and aging.

Obviously, our goal is to help patients look and feel their best, but this requires a joint effort between doctor(s) and patient. The patient's part is to be receptive to information about positive change which, if properly managed, will maximize the doctor's effectiveness and the patient's results. Because physical appearance and health are inextricably linked, getting and keeping the body as healthy as possible and working to achieve and maintain positive emotional and mental conditions are vital parts of our jobs. The results of looking good and feeling good are increased because each plays off the other, and they combine to increase the patient's satisfaction and the doctor's sense of accomplishment.

For more information about nutrition, you can contact the National Center for Nutrition and Dietetics (800-366-1655) or the government-funded extension service of your county or state government.

How Do You Handle Success?

Have you ever noticed that when you set a goal and make progress that you feel absolutely terrific? Perhaps you lost a few pounds and the jeans you bought look terrific. Or maybe you've been exercising and finally your body begins to feel and look more toned. How do you feel? Encouraged? Motivated? Proud? Happy?

These positive feelings are the motivators that enhance your efforts. Education gives you the power to improve, and motivation builds results. Let's take a good look at how a very determined woman applied both education and motivation as the formula for success.

The following personal account is based on information gathered in an interview with one of our patients who was a chubby child, a self-conscious teenager and young adult, a determined thirty year old, and now, at 46, a very attractive, self-confident woman who appears younger than her age. She sought medical advice regarding cosmetic surgery for liposuction of the abdominal area, and she wanted to improve sun damage to her skin on several parts of her body. Yes, we helped her, but we also encouraged her to learn more about herself and to consult a nutritionist and an exercise therapist.

Margaret (Age 40)

I have never been fat — just pudgy — and only in certain places. This was especially annoying because my legs were very thin, but my upper body stored the excess fat. In clothes, I learned to be a master of disguise. Certain outfits allowed me to appear thin all over, but come spring or summer, I had a harder time covering up my problem areas. I always joked about walking to the neighborhood pool, purposefully armed with a large towel and beach bag which I held in front of my body to cover my rounded tummy. I just knew that as I walked by the crowd of people who knew me, someone would say, "Goodness, I never realized she was heavy."

Once I got to a suitable lounge chair, I would sit down quickly, but I still held my towel and bag in front of me — over my stomach — until I was fully reclined. My thinking was that my stomach looked much flatter when I was lying down. Guess what? It was.

Once I had reclined in a position that would make my tummy look flat, I would remain in that position for the entire afternoon — face up, lying on my back, burning my skin, and thinking that, although I was miserable, I had to get a tan in order to be beautiful, and I had to lie on my back to disguise the body I was embarrassed about. I would leave the pool sunburned — but only on one side because God forbid, I never rolled over for fear someone would see the bulges in my middle.

Today I laugh at these memories, but I can't forget or make light of the terrible insecurity I felt. I also know that I was not alone as a child and later as a teenager in hating my body and allowing that insecurity to stand between me and self-confidence. I was so caught up all those years in disliking things about myself, but

I never had the opportunity to learn how I could change the things that bothered me. I don't know whether people back in the fifties and sixties were ever taught about the possibilities of change. I know I wasn't.

Sometime in the sixties, a book entitled Our Bodies Ourselves *appeared, and I avidly read it cover to cover. I didn't realize what I found so interesting about that book until it dawned on me that its message was: You don't have to have a perfect body. You just need to understand your body and be good to it. Somehow I was hearing that message for the first time in my life, and it was a relief. Until then, my body was an enemy over which I had no control.*

As I look back on it, I reminded myself of the comic strip character Cathy who vacillates from one personal dilemma to another and from one insecurity to another. She is much more aware of what she doesn't have than what she has. Although the comic character is very funny, it's not so funny in real life when you're the one feeling frustrated and inferior, or out of control of your life.

Once I began to combine two simple philosophies, my life changed for the better. I began to learn about the cause-and-effect relationship of what I ate, or, in other words, what food was doing to my body, and I began to learn about the physics of exercise or how certain kinds of physical activity and exercise could change the contours of my figure.

At first, I concentrated on gaining information and knowledge rather than on pressuring myself to start a specific program or make any drastic changes. I found that as I learned about the foods I was eating and got new insights into exercise, I actually changed my mind before I ever began to change my body. What I mean is that I changed the way I looked at things because I was armed with information. No longer was I simply responding and making emotional decisions.

The old saying that education is permanent and motivation is only temporary is so true because if you simply psych yourself up for a diet, you have to re-psych yourself constantly in order not to falter. But if you're deciding what to eat and how to exercise because you understand what's happening within your body, then your chances of success are much greater. I really believe that if you're trying to get somewhere in self-improvement, you have to work on your mind first.

I went to see a nutritionist who taught me about the best foods for me to eat in order to reduce the amount of body fat that I was storing away. I learned to eat different foods, and not only to eat them but to like them. For a person who used to eat mostly hamburgers, french fries, and sweets and who definitely ate out of boredom while I sat watching TV, I made changes that I never thought I'd even consider making. I not only made changes, I have come to prefer the different foods I eat today. When I occasionally eat the kinds of food which I used to crave, I don't feel as good. When I eat a meal, I have conditioned myself to be aware of getting full. Today, one of the things I never want to happen is to overeat at a meal because feeling full — which I used to equate with satisfaction — now makes me uncomfortable and miserable.

I am not and have never been on a "diet," and I never go hungry. I eat several times a day — usually more than three times because I get hungry often — but I eat different foods than I used to, and I never want the quantity of food at any one time that I used to like. I also take vitamin supplements which my nutritionist recommends.

Considering how far I have come in both education and behavior modification compared to where I started years ago, I'm not surprised at what I'm about to say. I actually like my body, and I'm very proud of my figure. It's certainly one of my best features. Yes, I'm still a little vain, but I've definitely changed in other ways. I have realized what it means to respect my body, not just for how it can look but for how well prepared it is to get me through the rest of my life.

I can honestly say that I have enjoyed living in my body for the last 15 years, and more today even than five or so years ago. I am of normal weight for my 5'6" height — about 120 pounds — my percentage of body fat is on the healthy low side, and I have more strength and stamina than I did at age 18. I am very secure wearing a bathing suit, and I walk around the pool empty handed. I wear fitted clothes, and I no longer feel heavy and uncomfortable from the waist up or when I sit down.

How have I done it? I changed the way I look at food, and that changed my food preferences. Plus, I don't just pay attention to weight anymore. I watch my percentage of body fat, the number of fat grams eaten per day, blood pressure and cholesterol levels, etc. There are just a few basic numbers that I watch pretty closely because they are my safety gauges.

I also found out that physical activity doesn't have to be strenuous jogging in order to count. I've actually found an exercise program I enjoy and healthy foods I love to eat. That's important because I do still love to eat. That will probably never change.

Margaret's story is so clear. In order to eat smart, it is necessary to think smart. This means understanding what the body needs, learning why the body requires certain elements, and discovering how and why an attractive appearance, health, and longevity are linked to nutrition. Unfortunately, modern eating involves many fatty, empty calories which may provide temporary gratification; but they fail to provide important dietary elements which enable the body to operate efficiently, promote its resources and reserves, and keep running smoothly for many years ahead.

Once she understood that changes were possible and that they would not be that hard to make, she got very motivated — especially when she began to see results. The greatest part of her story is that she not only made some self-improvement changes, she changed her life in many ways, all for the better.

In the next section let's take a good look at what happens to the body when the aging process begins and learn how certain nutrients found in the foods we eat play a key role in that process.

Free Radicals

This sounds suspiciously like a political term from the sixties, but in fact free radicals are unstable molecules which play havoc with our bodies. They literally attack other unsuspecting molecules, setting up reactions that are damaging to healthy cells in the body. This damage is one of the major causes of the aging process. The "free radical theory of aging" deals with how nutrition can help counteract the effects of aging.

Richard A. Passwater, Ph.D., author of a best-selling book on health and vitality entitled *The New Super Nutrition,* calls free radicals "chemical terrorists," explaining that one free radical can damage a million or more molecules. Free radicals are capable of widespread destruction, and they indiscriminately attack various organs of the body. They are highly reactive molecular fragments which attack cell membranes and kill the active cell or change it to a cancer cell.

Examples of this process occur all around us. Everyone has seen fruits such as bananas or apples cut in half and left open exposed to the air. What happens? They turn dark and become shriveled. If left unrefrigerated, dairy products will spoil and turn sour. And here's an unpleasant thought. Even a soft, wrinkle-free baby's skin will turn coarse and weathered due to the free radicals' interaction with sunlight. Aging has been explained as a process during which the body's healthy cells are reduced. As we age, each organ of the body loses its own cells, reducing its reserves and ability to ward off further aging and disease. Thus, the damage caused by free radicals moving through the body, attacking and destroying cells, is clearly a major cause of the aging process.

Slowing Down the Aging Process

Researching free radicals at the University of Nebraska College of Medicine, Dr. Denham Harman sought the answer to the obvious question: What causes the free radical reaction in the human body? The answer he found is oxidation, the result of interaction between oxygen and matter. Free radicals cannot operate without oxygen. The fruit would not turn dark unless exposed to air.

Dr. Harman continued his research, seeking the answer to the next logical questions: How can the interaction of oxygen and matter be decreased without causing damage to the body's normal oxidation process, and how can the attack of free radicals on the body's healthy cells be decreased? The answers to these questions could unlock some of the mysteries still surrounding the aging process.

Dr. Harman's work, as well as research conducted by many other physicians and scientists who work in this field, has found answers in certain nutrients such as vitamin A, beta-carotene, vitamin C, vitamin E, and trace minerals and amino acids which, when ingested into the body, actually act as antioxidants. These antioxidants act as protection for the body from the destruction caused by oxygen interacting with matter.

As Dr. Harman points out, the antioxidants seem to have a "rust-proofing" effect within the body. Like treating metal so that it will not be destroyed, these antioxidants can help to protect the body from the aging process and are even believed to increase life expectancy.

The Miracle of Vitamin E

Dr. Harman also experimented with saturated and unsaturated fats. He conducted a study based on the theory that saturated fat causes an increase of cholesterol levels in the human body which can lead to atherosclerosis. In his study, Dr. Harman fed groups of mice and rats diets containing various amounts of unsaturated fats, 20 percent by weight of the total diet. Supposedly this experiment would show that these diets should have no difference on the mortality rates of the animals studied. Wrong. The group of mice who ate the greatest amounts of unsaturated fats had the highest mortality.

What this study revealed is that any high level of fat — even unsaturated fat — can decrease life span. The explanation is again linked to the destructive forces of free radicals within the body. Dr. Harman found that an increase of unsaturated fats increases the oxidation reaction in the body's cells, which speeds up the aging process.

Research shows that vitamin E — as well as many other vital nutrients — plays an important role in the anti-aging process. Dr. Harman found that feeding vitamin E to mice whose diets were high in unsaturated fats released the "rustproofing" effect which went to work fighting against free radicals. He also found that adding 20 International Units (I.U.) of vitamin E per 3.5 ounces of food reduced the number of breast tumors the mice tended to develop as the amounts of unsaturated fats were increased. Vitamin E also was found to increase the efficiency of their immune responses which increased their abilities to fight against infection.

Dr. Jeffrey Bland, a chemist at the University of Puget Sound in Washington who studied red blood cells in older people, also documented evidence that vitamin E is an important anti-aging factor. Dr. Bland found that red blood cells in older people take on a popcorn-like shape referred to as "budded" cells. According to his theory, this cell "budding" process is the result of oxidation damage to the cell membrane. In his experiments, Dr. Bland could actually make normal cells "bud" by exposing them to oxygen and air.

Dr. Bland studied the red blood cells of a group of donors who had been fed 600 I.U. of vitamin E every day for ten days prior to donating their blood. Interestingly, he found that exposing their blood to oxygen and air produced only a small number of cells which lost their shape. But when he exposed the blood of people who had not taken the vitamin E, their cells were totally transformed into "budded" cells.

Fat Facts

Recent scientific findings say that even the officially recommended diet guidelines may be too high in fat. The National Cholesterol Education Program (NCEP), a part of the National Institute of Health, has recommended that Americans limit daily fat intake to no more than 30 percent of total daily calories in order to reduce blood cholesterol. But many experts feel these guidelines do not go far enough in reducing fatal diseases associated with excessively fat diets typical of Western countries.

According to Colin Campbell, a nutritional biochemist at Cornell University, "The optimum level of fat intake is probably between 10 and 15 percent." However, surveys indicate the average adult in the United States includes about 37 percent of total calories from fat.

Dr. Campbell recently conducted a study of eating habits and lifestyles in isolated villages and towns throughout China. His study has produced the largest collection of data on disease, diet, and the environment, not to mention some interesting comparisons between Chinese and American diets:

• Chinese people consume 20 percent more calories than Americans, yet Americans are 25 percent fatter. Chinese eat only one-third the amount of fat that Americans do, and Chinese eat twice the amount of starch Americans do.

• A protein-rich diet — especially a diet heavy in animal protein — is linked to chronic disease. Americans consume one-third more protein than Chinese people do, and 70 percent of the protein in American diets comes from animal sources, while only 7 percent of the Chinese diet comes from animal sources.

• Childhood diets high in calories, protein, calcium, and fat promote growth and early menarche (the first menstrual period) and are associated with high cancer rates. A rich diet which promotes rapid, early growth in life may increase a woman's risk of developing cancer of the reproductive organs and the breast.

• Dairy calcium is not needed to prevent osteoporosis. Most Chinese consume no dairy products and get their calcium intake from vegetables. Chinese calcium consumption is only half that of Americans, yet osteoporosis is uncommon among Chinese people.

However, Chinese people living in the United States who develop American eating habits also develop our heart-disease patterns.

Research also shows that most people are unaware of the types of fat they consume and that education usually comes only after a problem has occurred. It is much easier to control fats in the diet before a health problem occurs, and limiting fats — especially animal fats — does not mean going on a bland, boring diet. In order to begin to clear up some of the confusion, here are some valuable fat facts.

Fat has more than twice the amount of calories as protein or carbohydrates. The most dangerous kinds of fat come from animal and dairy sources, but the way in which fats are formed or processed play an important role too. Getting the fat facts straight has some people rather confused, but it's actually very simple. The main types of fat which concern us are saturated fats, polyunsaturated fats, and hydrogenated fats. Each type consists of carbon, hydrogen, and oxygen in various combinations.

Saturated fat gets its name from its construction, allowing the fat to contain all the hydrogen it possibly can. A saturated fat is easily recognizable because it is solid at room temperature.

Polyunsaturated fat is not filled to capacity with hydrogen, but its carbon molecules do contain more than one (poly) hydrogen atom. Polyunsaturated fat is also easily identified because it is liquid at room temperature.

Hydrogenated fat gets its name from the process that manufacturers use to turn a liquid fat (corn oil) into a solid fat (Crisco) by chemically adding hydrogen to the liquid. This process changes the fatty acids, increasing saturation levels and altering some of the natural components into unnatural arrangements. The hydrogenation process can create an abnormal type of fatty acid which can collect in the heart and cause problems.

Generally speaking, the large body of research indicates that it is best to limit saturated fats in the diet because saturated fats are not healthy for your heart. Some studies show that substituting polyunsaturated fats for saturated fats reduces cholesterol and lowers the risk of heart disease. Research also tells us that limiting the amount of fat in the diet to the newly established lowered levels and limiting the amount of fat consumed from animal sources is the healthiest heart advice. Just keep in mind that fat, no matter what its makeup, is fattening — about 100 calories per tablespoon.

Dietary Fats

Here's a quiz from the American Heart Association:

True or False:
1. A 3-ounce portion of meat is about the size of a compact disc.
2. When the desire for high-fat desserts overtakes you, you should eat fruit and try to forget the urge for sweets.
3. If a food product label says "no cholesterol," you can feel safe eating it.
4. Even if your blood cholesterol is in the desirable range (less than 200 mg/dl), it's smart to have it checked every five years.
5. It's OK to eat all the polyunsaturated fat you want.
6. Non-dairy creamers are low in fat.
7. Skim milk is best for most adults — but not for babies.
8. Lowering your blood cholesterol from 250 to 200 mg/dl may reduce your risk of heart attack by 40 percent.
9. Saturated fat is found only in products of animal origin.

Answers:
1. **False.** It's the size of a deck of cards.
2. **False.** You may eat a small serving or share it with a dining partner. Occasional sweets are OK in moderation in proportion to a well-balanced diet.
3. **False.** A product without cholesterol may contain saturated fat, which raises blood cholesterol. Read labels carefully for the kind of fat listed.
4. **True.** This is what the American Heart Association recommends.
5. **False.** Polyunsaturated fat can decrease blood cholesterol, but it's not known whether large amounts of polyunsaturated fat are safe. The AHA recommends a fat intake of up to 10 percent of your total calories.
6. **False.** Non-dairy creamers are loaded with saturated fat. Instead, opt for 2 percent milk or skim milk.
7. **True.** Skim milk is best for adults. But babies need the fat in breast milk formula or whole milk at least until age two.
8. **True.** For every 1 percent your blood cholesterol is lowered, your risk of heart attack death may be reduced by 2 percent.
9. **False.** Saturated fat is also found in vegetable sources. Coconut and palm kernel oil are particularly high in saturated fat. Cholesterol is found only in products of animal origin.

Sometimes it is hard to know just how fat fat is because many product labels are misleading, and many foods you order are improperly named. For instance, the formula "percent fat free" is based on the weight of the product. While a product may be only 10 percent fat by weight, forty to fifty of the calories could come from fat. The Food and Drug Administration is working to improve labeling requirements. The best advice is to start questioning what you're eating and to match your consumption to healthy guidelines.

Saturated Fats

Conservative advice is to limit your intake of saturated fats to no more than 10 percent of your total calories. Saturated fats cause the cholesterol plant in your liver to increase its output, which raises your blood cholesterol level and increases risk of heart disease. Saturated fats come from sources such as beef, pork, lamb, veal, egg yolks, whole milk, cream, cheese, ice cream, butter, chocolate, coconuts, and fats that are used in the processing of many foods such as palm oil and coconut oil.

Fat Formula

In order to determine the percentages of calories from fat, use this formula below:

Unsaturated Fats

The fats known as polyunsaturated and monounsaturated fats slow down the liver's cholesterol output and lower your blood cholesterol level. But you still have to watch your intake of them because calorie-wise, these fats are worth about 100 calories per tablespoon. Unsaturated fat sources are plant foods such as vegetables, grains, seeds, nuts, fruits, beans, and the oils derived from these sources. A "no cholesterol" label really means that the plant sources are naturally cholesterol free.

Cholesterol

We hear so much about cholesterol, but what is it anyway? Simply put, cholesterol is a fatty substance which is found in all animal tissues. It makes up

Grams of fat per serving	X 9 =	Total fat calories per serving	÷	Total calories per serving	=	Percentage of calories from fat

A gram of fat contains nine calories. Multiply the grams of fat by 9 to get the number of calories. Divide by the calories per serving to get the percent of calories from fat.

an important part of the membranes of each cell in the human body, and we use cholesterol in many positive ways. The liver uses cholesterol to make bile acids which aid in digestion. The body uses cholesterol in the production of certain hormones, including the sex hormones.

Our bodies manufacture most cholesterol in the liver. There are special carrier molecules called lipoproteins which transport cholesterol out of the liver through the bloodstream to the various cells throughout the body. Lipoproteins come in three different types: the high-density lipoproteins, or HDL; the low-density lipoproteins, or LDL; and the very low density lipoproteins, or VLDL. This information is important to know because when your blood cholesterol levels are measured, they are identified by each type of lipoprotein carrying it through the body.

Although the body needs certain amounts of cholesterol to be healthy, high levels of certain types have been linked to increased risks of some diseases. Doctors generally suggest limiting cholesterol intake in order to manage optimum levels. While we manufacture most of our own, some extra cholesterol makes its way inside our bodies through animal food sources. Your blood cholesterol level goes up when you eat more cholesterol than the body can use. The foods which are the most common high cholesterol sources are egg yolks, the fat layer of dairy products such as whole milk and cream and the muscle portion of poultry and meats.

How cholesterol is measured is a very important part of the health picture. For example, most medical experts agree that, in general, the risk of heart disease is less if your cholesterol is under 200. This information represents only a general guideline for cholesterol — not the total picture. About 20 percent of heart attacks occur in people who have cholesterol levels under 200. The important thing to understand is how to interpret a total cholesterol level; the doctor must determine HDL as well as LDL levels because each type plays a different role.

Cholesterol Questions and Answers

1.   How high should HDL cholesterol be?

Your total cholesterol divided by your HDL level should ideally be under 3.5.

2.   What does excess cholesterol mean?

When your total cholesterol is over 150 or when your LDL cholesterol is over 90, you have more cholesterol than the body can use. The body makes cholesterol and gets more cholesterol from food sources. When the cells in the body have more cholesterol than they can use, the excess begins to store away as waxy deposits that literally choke the cells. The only way the body can get rid of the excess is for the HDL (carrier molecules) to pick it up and carry it to the liver, where about 95 percent of it can leave the body as waste. The job performed by the HDL earns it the nickname "good cholesterol."

3. How does the cholesterol level help predict heart disease?

Most heart attacks occur in people with total cholesterol levels between 200 and 240. The LDL is a better predictor of heart disease than total cholesterol — even when the total is over 240 — because very few people have enough HDL to get them out of a high LDL — level problem.

4. What about triglycerides?

Triglycerides are the break-down products of cholesterol transported through the blood primarily by the very low density lipoproteins, or VLDLs. There is a debate about triglycerides, but studies show that they are often good predictors of heart disease. Triglycerides should be under 150.

5. How does exercise affect cholesterol levels?

Exercise is a wonderful way to stay in shape and keep trim, and it also helps raise the HDL and lower the LDL in healthy ratios. For healthy hearts, the biggest benefit comes in the first 2,000 calories used up in a week's time. About 500 calories is what a dedicated couch potato uses up per week. So, most of us are faced with finding pleasant ways to use up about 1,500 calories from exercise each week. If you walk briskly or jog, you use about 100 calories per mile. A successful schedule would break down to walking or jogging about 2 miles a day, which comes to 200 calories a day for seven days. That comes to 1,400 calories, which seems very "doable" for most people. If you want to burn up 200 calories a day in other ways, you can swim 800 yards, bicycle 5 miles, do aerobics for 30 minutes, run on a treadmill for 25 minutes, or row for 1.5 miles. Just keep the magic number of 2,000 calories per week in your mind, and work against that figure as your goal for a healthy heart.

Butter, Margarine, or Oil

When we think of healthy cooking and eating habits, many of us wonder whether to use butter, margarine, or oil. The bottom line is to use less fat. When you cook with or eat fat, go for the unsaturated oil choice. Margarine has less fat than butter, and the softer margarine found in diet tubs are lowest in calories. Butter, of course, is the last choice because it is highest in fats.

Fat from Meat

In order to count fats in meat, here's a chart to guide you.

MEAT	CALORIES	FAT (G)	% OF CALORIES FROM FAT
Eye of round, select	178	6	30
Chuck, select	222	9	36
Tenderloin, select	208	10	43
Chicken breast, skinless	165	4	21
Chicken breast, with skin	197	8	36
Chicken wing, with skin	290	19	59
Leg of Lamb	191	8	38
Pork tenderloin	166	5	27
Ham	220	11	45
Turkey breast, skinless	135	1	7
Turkey breast, with skin	153	3	18
Shoulder roast of veal	170	7	37

(Values are for 3.5 ounces of cooked and well-trimmed meat.)
Source: *University of California at Berkeley Wellness Letter*, August 1991

The fifth edition of the *American Heart Association Cookbook* (Time-Life Books) contains updated information about the effects of diet on heart disease, cancer, and other diseases, as well as guidelines for reading food labels, adapting favorite recipes to low-fat cooking, and many ideas which support the fact that healthy eating does not have to mean deprivation and unsatisfying foods.

Drink Water and Stay Young

These days it is increasingly popular to drink water and especially bottled water, which is thought to be purer than plain tap water. Many of us are giving up diet drinks which are generally high in caffeine and chemicals and quenching our thirsts with water. As a matter of fact, drinking plenty of good, clean water is as important to the human body as getting the right nutrients from food or dietary supplements. We're holding fast to the recommendation that eight glasses of water per day is a good prescription for health.

Most of us already know that the human body is made up of about 98 percent water. The reason why water is so important to the body's health is because water ensures the body's natural balance. We lose water each day through elimination, perspiration, respiration, and exercise. If you do not replace the water that is lost, the body becomes unbalanced, and many of the biological processes which regulate the body, such as body temperature, blood pressure, and respiration, are affected. Bodily functions depend on an adequate water supply in order to work and function properly and to maintain the ability to function well as the body ages. Water allows the body to excrete waste products it would otherwise accumulate.

Look at the kidneys, for example. They perform the vital function of eliminating waste and controlling the body's internal water balance. Like other organs, the kidneys perform their jobs very well in healthy, normal, young people. However as people age, their kidneys are increasingly sensitive to changes in the body's intake of fluids and are not as efficient with waste elimination. The regulatory mechanism of the kidneys is just not as efficient as it used to be.

In addition, as we age we actually have a lower rate of sweating because it takes more to make us sweat than it used to. Perspiration, like the function of the kidneys, also plays an important part in the body's waste elimination process. Medical experts tend to agree that as we age, drinking adequate amounts of water combined with regular exercise (as addressed above) can actually improve the body's ability to regulate its internal temperature and maintain efficient waste elimination.

Like so many interesting facts about the human body, healthful conditions are always the result of a combination of factors. No one component stands alone in producing or maintaining health. We encourage you to read and learn as much as possible about the human body and about what makes it function well. Your education about your body and health is the greatest motivating factor in your lifelong journey to be your best.

The WIIFM Theory of Health Management

Too often we know what we should and should not do in order to maintain health. We hear "lower fat intake," "take your vitamins," "drink plenty of water," but in order to be motivated to take the right steps, you need to understand why. Every time you read or hear medical or health advice, apply the WIIFM theory of health management. This means asking "What's in it for me?" This is not an selfish question but a practical one, and the answer may be just the motivating factor you need to understand and initiate positive changes. After all, when we understand the whys and hows and relate that information to our own bodies, we are much more likely to succeed in whatever self-improvement steps we decide to take — from eating smart to shaping up, which is the subject of the next chapter. We are not nutritionists or experts in exercise, but we know that without these two major health components, most medical treatments and procedures cannot be fully utilized and that all the beauty tricks and fashion statements in the world are mere temporary gratifications. We also know that nutrition and exercise set the foundation for all other self-improvement goals and in large part enhance their results.

This is why we are such strong advocates of healthy nutrition and exercise. We encourage our patients to seek council from reputable experts in these fields, to educate themselves by reading books and articles on the subjects, to realize that the proper combination of nutrients can prolong a healthy life, and to get their whole family into a routine of eating smart. Regardless of age, what you eat today in large part determines how you will look and feel in the future.

THE FITNESS FACTOR

In this chapter we present various fitness formulas for improving personal fitness. There are many different effective ways to achieve physical fitness, and no one method is perfect for everybody. Also, individuals like variety in exercise programs in order to maintain interest in exercising and to balance long-term results.

We will also discuss some very interesting reasons why fitness is an important factor in the anti-aging and quality-of-life campaign. We'll begin with a close look at the "triggers" which motivate people to exercise or work out. Exercise triggers are as important as the appetite triggers we discussed in the preceding chapter. Finding out what motivates you to exercise is key to success.

All the Right Reasons

In an informal survey of our patients, we asked a number of men and women who exercise regularly to identify their motivating factors. Of course, many of their answers involved weight control, but the majority said that though weight control was a great by-product of exercise, other motivating factors were more significant.

Over 85 percent of the people we questioned, whose ages ranged from 18 to over 65, said they exercised for this reason: "Because exercise made them look and feel better." Other answers included the responses listed below. As you read these responses, ask yourself, "What is my motivation for exercise, or what would it be if I were to begin an exercise program?"

- "Exercise gives me a high that I cannot get from anything else."

- "I work out because I am very competitive. I compete against others, and I compete against the goals I set for myself."

- "My job is very sedentary. If I didn't exercise, I'd never move around much at all."

- "Exercise helps me sleep better and slows down my appetite — especially if I exercise in the evening, which is when I get the munchies."

- "I get very anxious and nervous. Exercise is the only thing that really helps me improve my self-control. You could say that exercise is my attitude adjuster."

- "I want to keep my body young looking and my muscles toned."

- "I am a very physical person. Aerobic and weight training keeps me looking the way I want to look and helps me channel my energy in a very positive way. Plus, being involved with fitness helps me meet many people who think like I do."

- "I get headaches from tension and stress if I don't exercise."

- "Exercise gives me a great feeling of personal power. I make my own decisions when I'm exercising and I feel totally free."

The patients we interviewed are involved in various forms of exercise, from walking and running in parks or on treadmills to cross-training activities. They bike, golf, play racquet sports, do yoga, hike, garden, attend aerobics and body-building classes, use weight training, dance, play team sports, do calisthenics, and swim.

Something for Everyone

The point is, there is an enjoyable exercise for anyone who is in good health and has a mind set to get started. The favorable reasons for regular exercise could take up a book of their own, but each person — regardless of age — needs to find an enjoyable exercise and get started right away. It will make you feel better and look better. It may even prolong your life.

There are two important points to remember: One, you should not begin any exercise or increase any level of exercise without consulting your doctor to be sure your plan is appropriate for you; and two, all exercise should be viewed with the positive end results in mind.

Do not be misled into thinking that when it comes to exercise, there are only two kinds of people: those who like exercising and those who do not. The truth is that most people do not think they like exercise at all until they practice it regularly for an extended period of time. Then most people who have been exercising regularly for an extended period say they learn to enjoy it. First and foremost, people like the results they get; exercise firms the body and helps build stronger muscles and bones. It also controls weight, increases strength and flexibility, quickens the mind, increases relaxation, decreases stress, and enhances self-image.

Second, people learn to like exercise because they say it gives them a natural high they cannot get from any other source. People who learn to exercise regularly even claim they have a hard time going without it because they are addicted to the exhilarated feeling they get after a good exercise session.

Researchers at the University of California at Berkeley point out that a primary reason why exercise makes people look and feel better is because these people tend to have healthier hearts. What happens is that when the heart pumps blood throughout the body, each cell is nourished with oxygen. People who exercise regularly improve the ability of their hearts to pump blood throughout their bodies and to better nourish the cells with oxygen. This is also why people who exercise are said to have a "glow."

Exercise is the best thing known to help keep the heart working efficiently, the muscles strong, and the body toned throughout the years. It also reduces the risk of diseases such as diabetes and heart disease and has a rejuvenating effect on body organs. Exercise is linked to a decrease in depression and an increase in personal happiness and is credited with giving people an added feeling of vigor and vitality. New research suggests that regular aerobic exercise even leads to an increased interest in sexual activity.

David P. McWhirter, M.D., at the University of California at San Diego studied a group of healthy but sedentary men who ranged in age from 36 to 65. These men started riding stationary bikes or jogging every other day for one hour. After nine months, the men reported they were experiencing increased sexual activity — three times a week or more on the average, which represents a 30 percent increase since they began exercising. They also reported an increase in sexual fantasy and sexual enjoyment, as well as an increase in self-esteem, which was no doubt linked to the better body images they developed as a result of the nine-month program.

Exercise is increasingly important after age 25 or so, when the first signs of physical change begin to occur. For many people weight control becomes more difficult even though eating habits and caloric intake may not have changed. Many find that each year unchecked pounds tend to mount, and fat starts to accumulate in telltale places. Also, research shows that after age 25, the rate at which the body processes and delivers oxygen declines about 1 percent per year and that even youthful people who do not use muscles lose the optimal functions of those muscles.

In the weight-control arena, the physical changes for both sexes are predictable. In women, fat usually clings to hips, thighs, and buttocks or collects in the abdomen and midriff area. Men tend to collect deposits of fat in the abdomen, through the waist and under the chin. As a rule, women have a tendency to gain excess fat in their lower bodies, and men have problems with excess fat in their upper bodies. However, this very general statement has many exceptions; where you collect fat is unique to your individual body type and is largely determined by heredity.

Which Body Type Are You?

People with more fat in their upper bodies are referred to as having the "android" fat distribution pattern, and people with more fat in the lower body have what is called the "gynecoid" fat distribution pattern. Knowing your body type is important in determining an individual exercise plan which incorporates specific exercises that are effective in reducing body fat and toning particular problem areas.

Your body type is also an indicator of health risks. Studies show that the risk of certain diseases is affected by how much you weigh and where excess weight is stored. In general, the risk for disease and decreased life expectancy is higher for people with "android" fat patterns than it is for those with "gynecoid" fat patterns. This information applies even to people who are relatively thin.

In numerous studies over the years, men and women who have increased abdominal fat have been found to have a higher incidence of hypertension or high blood pressure, elevated lipids or fats, and an increase in diabetes. Obese women and women who have a high percentage of body fat have been found to have a greater risk of developing

breast cancer than those who are trim and have a low percentage of body fat. Women who have android fat distribution patterns have an increased risk of developing breast cancer than women with gynecoid fat distribution patterns. The reason for this difference has been linked to different hormone patterns in the blood of the two types of women. These risk-related statistics, like many other medical-risk predictions, can be offset, and the actual risk of disease can by decreased with a combination of proper nutrition, regular exercise, and, as needed, medical advice and treatment.

As those of you know who have tried to diet and exercise in order to get rid of weight from a specific area of the body, it is a very difficult process. We have patients who tell us that, try as they may, they cannot lose weight from certain areas such as in the "saddlebag" area at the outer thighs and in the "love handle" area around the waist. The most effective step is to begin a sensible, low-fat diet combined with aerobic activity and a recommended weight-resistance program designed to target the spot reduction desired. If you lose weight too fast, you will lose it in all the wrong places, and the weight will most likely come right back once you increase caloric intake. A very low calorie diet and the absence of a fitness routine is a terrible combination. If you do not combine exercise with proper nutrition, you will lose muscle faster than you will lose fat. What results is not a pretty sight — you will be left with flabby, excess skin where fat and muscle used to be.

You will look wrinkled and aged beyond your years.

And for those of you who want to try the rub-away creams which promise to break up fatty deposits and remove cellulite, save your money. Cellulite consists of fat-engorged cells that pull on the connective tissue holding them in place within the body. Cellulite is what causes those rippling dimples of fat that are hard to lose. The only way to get rid of cellulite is to lose the fat that fills the cells. Creams do not work — no matter how hard you rub.

In certain cases where diet and exercise have failed to produce the desired result in correcting a spot problem, the cosmetic surgical procedure called liposuction or lipolysis can be used. For example, if a woman has "saddlebags" at the outer thighs and she has found that diet and exercise improve the overall body but fail to improve her thighs, she may consider liposuction as a next-step option. If a man who has reduced weight and percentage of body fat and exercised routinely finds he cannot get rid of the fat that has collected in his abdomen, he may also consider liposuction. The chapter on cosmetic surgical procedures offers a detailed discussion on liposuction, which, when properly performed, is an effective procedure for enhancing body contours and improving spot problems in a woman's figure or a man's physique. Liposuction is not, however, a substitute for a smart nutrition plan or healthy exercise.

A Smart Plan for Your Future

The best all-around solution is to establish both a nutrition and exercise plan which are designed just for you. Regardless of your present weight or age, you need certain nutrients to improve and maintain your health and keep you young longer.

Just as you make a financial plan and buy health insurance, your nutrition and exercise plan paves the way for many secure, healthy, active years ahead. Don't be caught short, getting down the road and wishing you had done things differently or made changes earlier in life. Take steps right away to plan for your future.

The key factors to consider in establishing a nutrition and exercise plan are your age, sex, body type, percentage of body fat, exercise habits, height, and current weight. Heredity factors and your family's incidence of diseases such as heart disease, cancer, and diabetes are also important. Both a nutrition and exercise plan should be designed around these factors and selected to match your personal preferences as often as possible.

As you learned in the preceding chapter, nutrients and combinations of nutrients can be used effectively to control factors which are potentially damaging to body functions. After consulting your doctor, you may consider consulting an expert in the field of nutrition who can help you tailor an eating plan to your needs and lifestyle. A smart eating plan will augment your exercise program because it can help balance your caloric intake against your degree of physical activity. It can also help you understand what foods to eat in order to get the right amounts of protein and carbohydrates for your age, weight, and activity level.

A visit with a nutritionist can teach you what you need to know about foods, food preparation, and nutritional supplements. You'll also learn what to eat at home or in restaurants that will taste good and keep you from feeling hungry or deprived. Keep in mind that exercise should not be used to compensate for overeating or eating the wrong foods. A good nutrition plan maximizes an exercise plan, and if the two are planned together, your work will be much easier.

A nutrition plan does not have to be a rigid routine of tasteless foods. It basically helps you understand the best food groups from which to select, what foods to avoid, and how much to eat in order to balance your diet. An exercise plan does not have to be a boring or grueling schedule that you feel forced to follow. It is a simple road map that leads you along the path you've chosen for looking and feeling fit. As we said, it may be helpful to approach healthy eating and fitness in much the same way as you make a financial plan for the future. After all, isn't the purpose of a financial plan to prepare for the future, to build reserves for a day when you may not have as many resources at your fingertips, and to plan for your future life? The investment you make in your body is also a very important part of your plan for the future.

Follow Your Heart

If you slow down or stop exercising when your body gets tired, you may not be working your heart rate up into what is referred to as the aerobic zone. Most exercise experts define the aerobic zone as a heart rate of 70 percent of its maximum beats per minute. When your heart rate is raised by consistent, regular aerobic exercise, the real benefits of this kind of conditioning begin to kick in: improved cholesterol levels, lowered blood pressure, reduced body fat, and cardiovascular conditioning.

Your doctor will be able to help you determine how much exertion is needed to put you into the aerobic zone. Age, fitness level, and degree of exercise difficulty should be considered, and you can find your aerobic-zone heart rate by using the formula in the following example: An average woman at age 40 would subtract her age from 220. This figure, 180, is her maximum heart rate. Seventy percent of 180 is 126, her target heart rate for aerobic exercise. To work her heart up to 126 beats a minute requires brisk — but not intense — exercise. Most likely she could reach the desired rate by walking one mile in 15 minutes, for example.

Now, let's look at different exercise options to find one that is just right for you. If you're already exercising regularly, please read on because the next several pages contain new ideas about exercises you may want to try, interesting facts about how exercise works on the body, and some WIIFM advice about fitness.

Designing Exercise

Generally speaking, in order to be fit, you need to exercise at least three times a week for thirty minutes each session at 70 percent of your maximum heart rate. If you want to lose extra weight or reduce body-fat percentage, you need to increase the frequency and duration of exercise, but the intensity — which is measured by the heart-rate percentage — can stay the same. The time spent exercising beyond the thirty-minute point is when the fat really starts to burn off; during the first thirty minutes of exercise the body uses up carbohydrates in your blood stream, and after that it starts to use fat.

Today experts agree that moderate but frequent exercise is ideal, as opposed to the extremes of high-intensity and marathon exercise which is usually too rigorous for the average person. Besides, it is just as effective to maintain the frequency and duration of exercise and keep the intensity at a moderate pace. The most important personal consideration is to design exercise that will be challenging, enjoyable, and not so difficult that you burn out and quit.

Many people today join health clubs, attend exercise classes, hire personal trainers, and put together home gyms. These facilities and resources can provide excellent support for both mind and body. For people who like to exercise at home, consider turning a spare room, garage, or loft into an exercise facility. Some people install state-of-the-art weight-training and conditioning equipment; others outfit an exercise area on a very moderate budget. All across the country, there are excellent facilities with trained instructors at the YMCA/YWCA and YMHA/YWHA. They have equipment, offer classes and counseling, and, in many cases, provide child care. These organizations are nonprofit, and many offer financial aid.

For people who prefer the privacy of exercising at home and do not want to invest much money, try something like this: Buy a small round indoor trampoline. (The type with removable legs can slide under a bed and should cost no more than $25.) Turn on the radio or your favorite dance tapes (most cassette tapes are about 15 minutes per side), and run in place or do aerobic dance steps on the trampoline for workouts of about 30 to 45 minutes. You can also do this exercise while you're watching the morning or evening news or during a favorite television show. As you progress with this routine, try using light ankle and wrist weights to add small amounts of resistance to the aerobic workout. This kind of exercise is fun, offers a great workout, and is a low-impact aerobic activity. Low-impact aerobics gives you sufficient cardiovascular stimulation without the musculo-skeletal stress of jogging on the street or a track. Plus, running or dancing on the trampoline is easy on feet and legs and is less stressful to the back than high-impact exercises.

For people who do not like jogging or attending aerobic classes, the trampoline is great, and it is certainly an inexpensive alternative to other exercise options requiring club memberships or costly equipment. Once you have become accustomed to this activity, you may choose to add some additional weight-training exercises designed to firm and tone your body.

Step Up and Strengthen Your Heart

Another aerobic exercise that is very popular and effective is called stair-stepping or bench-stepping, which involves stepping on and off a low bench or stair step to music. This is a very efficient exercise because it builds muscles and burns up calories at the same time. There are step classes offered at health and exercise clubs which range in levels of ability and endurance, but you can also stair-step at home by building a simple bench-like step that is between 4 and 12 inches high, or you can use the first step of a staircase.

You can also purchase a ready-made step which is available in varying heights. The different heights are used to increase or decrease intensity as skill and ability vary and progress. As you add additional height to the step, you increase your oxygen consumption which is a good indication of how hard the body is working. The idea behind the stair-step exercise is to accomplish sufficient cardiovascular stimulation and, at the same time, build muscle tone and strength. Experts say this exercise is an excellent high-intensity, low-impact activity that is good for the heart.

The step can be tough on your knees though, so be sure that as you step up, you place your foot flat on the step or bench, and do not bend your knees any more than you would climbing regular stairs. Pay attention to correct posture: keep your back straight and avoid letting your body lean over when you step. Keep the choreography simple and repetitive, and if you change the speed or rhythm of the music, do so gradually, building up to faster speeds and more intensity with added practice. Be sure you have a good pair of shoes that provide proper support for this kind of activity.

The step exercise is a favorite with many people, and it does not seem to be too strenuous for most people who are accustomed to doing some degree of aerobic exercise. The main idea is to start slowly and build up gradually. Remember to see your doctor before starting any exercise program.

Success Stimulators

A major component of exercise success is understanding your present self-image and envisioning yourself as you would like to be. The term *visualization* refers to the images you see in your mind. For instance, if you are very hungry you can visualize certain foods that would taste wonderful. If you visualize this image strongly enough, you may find yourself on the road ordering the dish or buying the ingredients to make it.

Because mental programming is an important part of achieving objectives, visualization techniques can work very effectively in helping you make the exercise-nutrition connection. Research supports the theory that people who can see themselves in a specific environment, or who can envision how a change will make them look and feel, have a better chance of getting there. Look at it this way: If you can visualize yourself at a targeted weight, with improved muscular definition, or with a shapelier figure in a new bathing suit, you will be much closer to making it happen than if you simply said, "I wish I could lose weight and shape up."

That's why buying an article of clothing such as a bathing suit when you first begin a weight loss/fitness program and using it as a symbol of the goal you have set for yourself may be very helpful. As you work to turn your vision into reality — looking good in the bathing suit — you are constantly aware of the result you are striving for. You set measurable goals regarding weight loss and body-fat reduction, and you measure inches as you lose them. Then you try on the bathing suit every two weeks, for example, and visually mark your progress. The vision you have of yourself in that bathing suit can be very

motivating. It can help to keep you focused on your goal, boost your spirits if you get discouraged, and actually help you reach your goal faster.

The human mind has tremendous power, and like muscles, the mind can be trained and strengthened. Visualize yourself the way you want to be. As you progress toward your goals, pat yourself on the back, carefully mark your progress, and learn about the psychological and emotional motivators that drive you and help you win.

For example, what makes you want to keep exercising once you begin? This is a crucial question because "regular" exercise is what you need — not sporadic start-stops. Research shows that the best plans often go the way of the new running shoes or equipment which now sit somewhere in a dark closet waiting for another wave of enthusiasm to strike.

In order to stimulate your own success within any plan you set, it is important to acknowledge the good results you obtain as you progress. Create a measurement system, such as a simple desk calendar, pocket calendar, day planner, or diary where you log your feelings and document your progress as the days and weeks go by. Each day write a few simple phrases or sentences about how you feel, what you see, and how you look. Reread the records to see just how far you've come and to keep your motivation on track. The way clothes fit, the changing degree of body firmness and tone, the inches lost or gained, the shapelier figure, the healthy feeling, the exercise "glow," the enhanced sense of self-esteem — all these results will increase your motivation and push you toward your goals. The more you focus on how great you feel about your results, the more you will want to keep the program going. One day, you'll find that your program of healthy nutrition and exercise is merely a way of life.

No Pain, More Gain

The trick is to find an exercise activity that you're comfortable with and that doesn't seem too difficult or strenuous. If you haven't found a good marriage of exercise and enjoyment, keep trying different activities until one fits. There are many exercises to choose from, and one of them will "feel right" if you just experiment and find it.

Beginning a new exercise or weight-training program involves getting the answers to many questions such as, "How much exercise should I do? How often can I exercise? How should I increase the amount of exercise I do? Is this exercise appropriate for me?"

Qualified trainers and professionals at health clubs can help you answer these questions. There are numerous detailed books written by qualified experts in the fields of fitness and sports medicine which outline exercise programs and teach you about the equipment involved. But remember: consult your doctor first.

Exercise should not follow the old adage "no pain, no gain." Actually, the more we know about the benefits of exercise, the more we realize that you do not have to push hard or do high-impact aerobics in order to give your heart and muscles a good workout. Finding an exercise activity that suits you and that you can increase at intervals by adding more repetitions, speed, or intensity as you progress is crucial to long-term success.

There are several important elements which increase the chances of your successfully continuing to exercise. If possible, find an exercise companion — especially when starting a new activity. In addition to enjoying the companionship, most people tend to stick with the program when they schedule to meet with another person for exercise. Another great success stimulator is music. Regardless of the activity or length of time spent at it, many people enjoy exercising more frequently and stay at it longer if they listen to music they like at the same time. Music creates a rhythm for movement, occupies your mind, distracts you from clock-watching, and makes you feel good. (However, do be careful if you use head-sets while walking or running near automobiles; it is practically impossible to hear the roar of a vehicle over music that is being piped directly into your ears. Using head-sets while walking or running on trafficked roads has contributed to many injuries and deaths.)

Start Walking

Since there is absolutely no reason to put off until tomorrow what will make you better today, and since an exercise program does not have to be strenuous in order to count, why not start walking? Overall, walking is probably the most available exercise for most people. You can walk at lunch time, after dinner, with the dog or the family, at the park, at a track or indoor facility, or at a shopping mall in extreme weather conditions.

The beauty of walking is that it's easy and an excellent exercise for all ages. It takes little or no pre-training and a minimal investment. It's also very gentle on the body — doesn't leave you with the typical aches and pains associated with more strenuous exercises. All in all, walking is an exercise that most of us can relate to and are probably already doing to some extent. It uses the large muscles of your body (leg, back, shoulders, and buttocks) and provides many benefits to the body if practiced regularly. But most important, walking is aerobic — it exercises the heart.

Get a comfortable, supportive pair of shoes (make sure your toes can move around inside the shoes), and put protective reflectors on your clothing if you plan to walk at night. When you are walking outdoors, be sure to use sunscreen to protect your skin from sun damage and premature aging all year round.

How to Lose Twenty Pounds This Year

Walking helps control weight and — like other aerobic exercises — can help you lose excess pounds. Let's suppose you are the kind of person who has gone on many fad or crash diets and have lost and gained the same twenty pounds over the last several years. This year it is possible for you to walk off the weight and maintain a balanced diet at the same time.

For example, if you want to lose one pound, you will need to burn up 3,500 calories. If you walk at a speed of two miles per hour for one hour per day, you will burn up 200 calories each day. That adds up to 6,000 calories per month with a weight loss of 1.7 pounds or slightly over twenty pounds in a year's time. And if you speed up the pace at which you walk to three or four miles per hour, the energy expenditure and weight loss increase proportionately. In all cases, the more exercise you do, the more calories you use and the more fat you lose. Exercise helps *maintain* weight loss, and when combined with sensible eating habits, it helps eliminate the "yo-yo" effect of fad diets.

When you walk, start out gradually and build up to increased levels with regular walking. Make sure that you walk on your whole foot rather than putting too much emphasis on your toes, which can strain the ankles and calves. Good walking posture includes walking with head erect and eyes front, tummy tucked in, and arms swinging freely at your side.

It is best not to walk right after eating — and especially not very fast. Let your food settle before walking in order to avoid muscle cramps; but do not lie down or get too relaxed because you may get sleepy as a result of what happens in the digestive process. In order for the body to absorb the digested nutrients from the food you have just eaten, approximately 25 percent of your total blood volume is detoured away from the brain and muscles toward the stomach.

Michael Pollack, Ph.D., director of the cardiac rehabilitation program at Mount Sinai Medical Center in Milwaukee, conducted a study using sedentary middle-aged men who were put on a 20-week walking program of 40 minutes of walking 4 times per week, with a gradual increase in walking tempo from 2.5 miles to 3.25 miles per session. By the end of the experiment, all the participants showed a drop in their resting heart rates. This result means that each man improved his cardiovascular system's ability to function by increasing his ability to take in more oxygen and enabling more oxygen to reach the tissues of the body in a more efficient manner.

Note: Please be aware of personal safety. Walking on streets, roads, and highways can be very dangerous. Every year walkers, joggers, and bikers are injured and killed by automobiles. It is extremely difficult to protect the human body from the kinds of injuries sustained in pedestrian (and biking) accidents, so please avoid competition with automobiles where you exercise. Walking or running in residential neighborhoods may also put you into contact with very territorial dogs. We have treated many patients for dog bites obtained while jogging through neighborhoods. These injuries are very traumatic and can produce serious wounds and scars. Exercise in familiar, safe, and protected places.

Can You See Your Muscles?

Men and women admire varying degrees of well-toned, shapely bodies and sculptured-looking physiques, but many of us may not have seen our muscles in years. The old joke about not being able to see your toes may be amusing to a pregnant woman who has a good excuse, but how many of us can honestly say that when we look at our bodies, we can see our muscles?

Often people think that a regular weight-lifting program will lead to a muscular-looking body. This is only partly true. Lifting weights before losing fat puts the cart before the horse. You cannot see the definition and shape of a muscle if it is covered under a layer of fat.

Look at any average male or female body (35+ years old) which has not had the benefit of a combined program of nutrition, aerobic activity, and weight resistance. Perhaps you can see some muscle definition in the calves of the legs or in the arms, but generally speaking, there is little or no visible evidence of muscles on other parts of the body.

In order to bring muscles out of hiding, to shape them and see their definition, the ticket is a combination aerobic workout routine, weight-resistance program — such as those using weight machines, free weights, calisthenics — and a low-fat nutrition plan. As the body decreases its fat reserves through aerobics and low-fat foods, the muscles, which are being shaped and defined by weight-resistance training, will become visible.

You can increase your muscle definition and strength by gradually adding heavier weights for increased resistance. But weight workouts should not be done everyday. The American College of Sports Medicine recommends two weight workouts per week — using free weights or machines such as those found in health clubs — and 8 to 12 repetitions of 8 to 10 different exercises that work on all the major muscles.

How Do You Build Strong Bones?

Bones can get thinner with age, and like muscles, they need exercise to stay young. Impact exercises help keep bones strong, and most workouts aimed at strengthening muscles also work on bones. Walking works on leg and hip bones, and calisthenics work on bones in the area of the body that gets exercised. For instance, leg lifts work on leg bones and push-ups work on arm bones. If you are getting a good aerobic and muscular workout, your bones are benefiting too.

Scale-Watchers Beware

The story is told of the trim, young woman who, upon being advised that she had a high percentage of body fat, looked at the doctor and said, "But that's impossible. I'm not the least bit overweight." This incident is not at all unusual because most of us measure how "fat" we are by stepping on the scales. However, weighing in may be deceiving because muscle and the other lean tissues of the body weigh more than fat. This is why many scale-watchers are annoyed when their weight begins to rise as they are trimming down with regular exercise. The facts are that weight is not necessarily an accurate measurement of how much body fat you are carrying around. The correct approach is to measure the proportions of fat and lean tissue in the body.

Medical experts agree that health risks are not associated with weight so much as with fat. Fat is the health threat associated with heart disease, diabetes, hypertension, and certain kinds of cancer.

But just how much body fat should you have? Most medical experts say somewhere between 14 and 22 percent for men and 18 and 27 percent for women is appropriate. The American College of Sports Medicine recommends slightly lower percentages: 11 to 18 percent for men and 16 to 23 percent for women. There are some physicians who say that women can still be within the healthy range at around 30 percent, but the growing consensus in the medical community is toward the lower percentage figures. The danger signs are clear. Men are considered obese at 25 percent and women at 35 percent. The startling news is that according to statistics, one in seven Americans is within the obese percentage range.

The important question about body fat is, "How do I measure up?" Body fat tests are available in hospitals, some doctors' offices, weight-loss clinics, and health clubs. But like other tests and treatments, the answer you get is only as accurate as the process, equipment, and technician involved in the evaluation. There are various types of tests available — all of which are painless, relatively quick, and affordable. Most of the tests available offer a reasonable measurement of body fat when properly administered, but there are variables and inconsistencies, so be sure to consult your doctor about the best test available for you. If you find your percentage of body fat is too high, the next question to answer is, "What can I do to correct my body composition?"

Easy Does It

From overeating to overworking, one thing we're all capable of is overdoing. Believe it or not, people can actually exercise too much, overtrain, and cause harm to their bodies. You may not envision yourself as an exercise addict or a workout maniac. You may see yourself as the kind of person who doesn't like exercise at all. You may even be smiling and saying to yourself as you reach this page, "I can skip this part." But please read on because when you do begin to see results from exercise, you will probably find that exercise isn't so bad after all. When you begin to enjoy exercise and look forward to that time in your day when there is no phone ringing, no traffic jam, no deadline to meet, you will understand how exercise can be addicting. But as with all things, you should strive to maintain a balance.

The B Word

Balance. It's probably the healthiest word in the English language. You should seek the same kind of balance in a healthy eating or exercise plan as you do in managing a busy work schedule to have some quality time set aside for yourself. Without balance, many people go too far in one direction; they mistakenly believe more is better. Like the man who worked up to jogging ninety miles a week, only to end up with serious back and knee problems, certain people become overzealous and carry a good thing too far.

What Does It Take to Get Fit?

The American College of Sports Medicine has set minimum fitness guidelines of three 20- to 60-minute sessions of aerobics at 60 to 90 percent of your maximum heart rate, combined with two body-building/strength-training sessions per week. These are general guidelines used to define what it normally takes to attain and maintain fitness.

However, each person is unique in both degree of fitness and capacity for exercise, and it is therefore impossible to outline guidelines which pinpoint when to stop exercising or working out. Determining excessive amounts of exercise is based on both physical and psychological indicators and is always an individual matter.

The important thing to remember is the difference between challenging yourself to attain greater heights and pushing so hard that you could trigger an injury. If you are exercising or working out frequently and experiencing extreme tiredness, chronic muscle soreness, and recurrent injury, you are probably over-exercising and deteriorating your body without allowing adequate time for repair. The reason for starting exercise slowly and gradually increasing intensity is to prepare the body for the extra demands placed upon it. Exercise should not be associated with pain. Although technically speaking, exercise is a process of tearing down and building back up, the body must have time to rest and recover from each vigorous exercise session. This is why most exercise guidelines do not recommend strenuous daily workouts.

If you have even wondered why most professional baseball teams have so many pitchers, it is because one game alone extracts an incredible toll on a pitcher's body. He has to rest between games. Here is an athlete who has practiced and trained extensively for his job, yet when he performs in one game, he sits out for several days and gives his body time to recover and rebuild itself before he plays again. The team has many pitchers because they literally have to recycle them in and out of the games throughout the playing schedule.

Taking care of yourself and finding the right balance in your life means that sometimes you will have to be your own coach and counselor, your own manager and motivator, and certainly, the final judge of what you elect to do and how you will accomplish your targeted results. Just remember that there are no quick fixes or overnight results in nutrition, weight-loss, or fitness programs. The positive long-term results come from an education that leads to behavior modification. You are the best person to take charge of your program. After all, who knows you better than you know yourself?

Here are some tips to help you make your program work:

1. Select your plan carefully.

2. Expect improvement, not perfection.

3. Set realistic goals within realistic time tables.

4. Schedule time on your calendar for regular fitness.

5. Pace yourself, starting slowly and building intensity gradually.

6. Find a balance of healthy, satisfying nutrition.

7. Find a companion and share the commitment.

8. Stretch and do inhale/exhale breathing warm-ups before exercising in order to increase circulation to muscles, joints, and tendons.

9. Cool down at the end of exercising and working out with a static (held) stretching and inhale/exhale breathing routine.

10. Fight boredom with results-based goals, self-motivation techniques, and competition.

11. Focus your mind on the end results of both improved fitness and appearance.

12. Exercise before eating and eat less.

Fitness Factor Summary

- Fitness is a temporary achievement that cannot be maintained without consistent exercise. The goal is to attain fitness and to maintain it — rather than attain it, lose it, and regain it. Ideally, fitness begins in childhood and is maintained throughout each stage of life.

- Exercise sensibly, starting slowly and increasing gradually. Consult your doctor and find out what your resting heart rate is. Ask your doctor to determine at what level your heart rate should be raised in order to enter the aerobic zone. The efficiency of your heart during exercise is a key factor in any fitness program.

- Dress sensibly for exercise. The body needs to maintain its normal temperature during exercise. If the body is too heavily clothed, it cannot cool itself properly.

- Be regular and consistent with any exercise and fitness program. General guidelines are three to four aerobic sessions per week for 30 – 45 minutes each. Some experts suggest five aerobic sessions per week for 20 – 30 minutes each. Each person is different, and each fitness program varies. Consult your doctor for individual advice.

• Weekend athletes who exercise vigorously can harm their bodies if they are not conditioned and prepared.

• It is not possible to burn fat in spot areas of the body, but aerobic exercise coupled with a low-fat diet makes it possible to burn away stored fat from all areas of the body.

H APPY, HEALTHY, AND WISE

May you live all the days of your life.
—Jonathan Swift

Just what is it that makes people happy? Many people think that happiness is simply beyond their reach, that they just aren't the right kind of people to be happy. But psychologists tell us that people of all ages, at every level of the socio-economic chart, of every race, in every country, can be happy.

We used to base happiness on the level of success a person achieved relative to his or her aspirations. For instance, if someone aspired to live in a big, expensive house, wear designer clothes, and drive a luxury car, but had not achieved these goals, then the person was most likely unhappy.

This kind of shallow thinking has no place in our world today. Definitive research clearly points to entirely different criteria for analyzing who is happy, who is not, and what really makes people happy. We know for sure that owning the big house, the great wardrobe, and the luxury car will not necessarily do the trick.

The consensus of research over the years seems to be that happiness — or "life satisfaction," as one psychologist terms it — stems from things we often overlook: interpersonal relationships among family and friends, communicating feelings and ideas comfortably and clearly, a feeling of control over one's life, and involvement in meaningful activity and new interests.

Go with the Flow

Many of us struggle with feeling out of control of our lives. "I have so much to do and so little time," we often say, or "I feel my life slipping by and soon it will be gone." Sometimes our minds wander back to simpler times, and we ask ourselves, "Gee, I wonder how life got to be like this? I didn't use to be in such a hurry."

Apparently being busy and stretched to the limit is not necessarily what makes people stressed out and unhappy. According to Mihaly Csikszentmihalyi, Ph.D., author of *Flow: The Psychology of Optimal Experience,* "Our best moments usually occur when a person's body or mind is stretched to its limits in a voluntary effort to accomplish something difficult and worthwhile."

Csikszentmihalyi contends that "each of us has thousands of opportunities to expand ourselves, but most of us waste our lives alternating between jobs we can't stand and leisure activities that offer little stimulation." His way of solving that problem is to create optimal experiences or "flow," which "lies in developing a mind that seeks new challenges and makes an effort to meet them." He adds, "When we find those areas for deep concentration, we forget ourselves and realize the most profound satisfaction."

The self-improvement changes discussed in this book simply help you take advantage of new opportunities for greater interest and increased satisfaction — to go beyond a boring job or unfulfilling leisure activities, to get off the couch or come out from behind the desk. Happiness *is* well within everyone's reach.

The Sandman

The longer you live, the more you know about life. Most people who have been around awhile readily agree that sleep is very important. Without sleep, it is pretty difficult to experience life's pleasures.

We all know what it's like to miss a good night's sleep from time to time, but it is important to be aware that cumulative sleep loss can affect both physical and mental health. A good night's sleep, however, is not necessarily the same for each of us. Some people can get by on as little as five or six hours of sleep a night. Some people even need as much as nine or more hours in order to feel rested, but the majority of us fall somewhere in the middle, requiring between seven and eight hours of sleep a night.

The amount of sleep we need does not decrease with age, as is often thought. In general, older people simply do not sleep as soundly as younger people. People of all ages can suffer insomnia, the chief cause of sleep loss. Insomnia and other sleep disorders tend to increase after age thirty, but there are several effective ways to combat the problem.

Insomnia is not a disease. Typically, it is an indication that something is bothering you — tension, stress, or certain aspects of your lifestyle. The goal for insomnia sufferers is to try to isolate the root of the problem and work on handling it so that relaxation and quality sleep can resume. It is important to find out what helps you relax and learn how you can turn off your mind so that you can fall asleep.

Some of the first indications that you may be suffering from a lack of sleep or quality sleep are frequent tiredness, a distracted mind, and sporadic loss of concentration, or you may feel irritable or depressed. One woman described exhaustion due to a lack of sleep as "when you start doing wild things like putting the coffee pot in the refrigerator or getting into the wrong car in a parking lot and wondering why your keys don't fit."

Everyone has insomnia occasionally. Perhaps you're worried about an important meeting, business problems, or financial problems. Maybe you have to catch an early-bird flight, and you're all wound up. Perhaps you hear noises in the house, and you feel anxious and afraid. The harder you try to sleep, the more sleep eludes you. Tossing and turning all night is awful, and most sleep experts agree that it does not help to try to sleep.

So what can you do? First of all, if insomnia has been a problem for two to three weeks at a time, see your doctor right away. Prolonged insomnia causes a breakdown in the body's precious reserves; is linked to an increased risk of infection, depression, and stress; and is considered to be both a medical and psychological problem.

Occasional insomnia is generally a temporary situation caused by stress or lifestyle. If you are worried about your job or anxious about making a presentation the next morning, you may toss and turn all night and be exhausted the next day. If you exercise at night or drink caffeine or alcohol, you may not be able to sleep. Even though an alcoholic drink may be referred to as a nightcap, the alcohol disrupts the stages of sleep and disturbs the quality of sleep. Nicotine is a stimulant which also keeps you awake, so here's one more reason not to smoke.

It is encouraging to know that the causes of occasional insomnia can usually be solved with some personal investigative work combined with a few steps in the right direction. The first thing to do is to identify any lifestyle factors involved in your sleepless patterns. These are the easiest areas to control and change.

For example, if you have trouble sleeping at night, avoid exercising in the evening; avoid stimulants such as alcohol, nicotine, and caffeine; try taking a nice leisurely bath, and always build in some time right before bed to wind down and relax. Create a routine of reading or watching the news on television, and do not save your problems to mull over after you are in bed. Establish a problem "cut-off time" (say, one hour before you go to bed), and do your best just to vegetate during this pre-bedtime period. Don't take phone calls, don't get involved in conversation, don't do any work, and don't think about stressful situations or problems.

Tune in your mind to the TV screen, some nice relaxing music, a good book, or a pleasant memory — whatever you enjoy that does not require a lot of brain power. As one man said, "I find it impossible to feel stressed when I'm watching reruns of old movies and television shows. I've seen them before, but I still like them. I think they relax me because when I'm watching them, I don't have to think."

In the case of stress- and anxiety-related insomnia, it is also necessary to identify what's bothering you — and to do something about it. We always hear only "Find out what's bothering you." The trouble is that many people find out or already know what's bothering them, but they don't take action and face the problem, eliminate it, or cope with it.

It has been said that it is impossible to focus on the problem if you are working on the solution. In cases of sleepless nights, most people who are working through their problems — confronting them, finding solutions, or just coping — sleep much better than those who are merely upset, anxious, depressed, or angry.

Real Solutions

No one wants to worry or be anxious, so here's a summary of some simple "feel better" examples and steps you can use to chase your troubles away, feel better all day, and sleep through the night.

• Many people dwell on their problems longer than they have to and — in view of their own emotional and physical health — experience them even more intensely than they should. Problems need to be identified and dealt with. If you are worried about a problem, the only solution is to confront the situation. When you do confront your problems with action rather than simply fretting over them, you will feel better, have greater peace of mind, and sleep better.

• Too often people worry about things they cannot control and suffer anxiety over situations that haven't even happened yet. Being anxious about what could happen down the road or worrying about things beyond your control is irrational behavior. It is also a source of anxiety that you can train yourself to curtail. Here's how one woman confused needless anxiety with real fear but began to take control of the very problem she worried about most.

I couldn't sleep at night and even worried about going home after work because I live alone and am afraid of intruders. I tossed and turned all night and hated staying alone. This may seem like a silly problem, but it was very real to me. I was losing sleep over it. Finally, I had to take some action. First, I got advice on how to best secure my doors and windows. Next, I contacted a local security company and had them install an electronic security system. I met with the security company representative who advised me of all my options. I decided to make my house as safe as I possibly could. Next, I signed up for a self-defense class. I learned several ways to increase my ability to defend myself should I ever have to do so.

Mostly, these lessons gave me a lot of confidence and a feeling of personal power. I used to feel defenseless — like I was just waiting for someone to break into my house and get me. Now I have a very different way of looking at this problem. Since I took action and began to take control of my personal security, I began to feel better. I also noticed that I began to sleep better too. As the weeks and months went by, I noticed that, although I was very cautious about security and always tried to protect myself, once I was inside the house and turned on my alarm, I was able to relax so much better, and I rarely had problems sleeping again.

- If you find that you tend to be anxious and fretful, even obsessed with problems, try to focus on positive "self-talk." Get control of your mind and make an effort to tell yourself the right things. Train your mind to think positively. Stop playing "what if" games with yourself. What if I get sick? What if I lose my job? What if I run out of money? These anxieties are unreal because the situations have not happened. If you play "what if" games, remind yourself that you are worrying about something that hasn't happened yet. If you have a problem or a real fear that concerns you, do everything you can to resolve it or keep it from happening, but be sure to focus on prevention rather than dwelling on anxiety.

- Experiencing stress, anger, and tension (SAT Syndrome) or harboring fear, uncertainty, and doubt (FUD Factor) are much tougher than taking active steps toward prevention or working through problems or unpleasant situations. And when you do, you'll probably find that you not only sleep better, but your entire life seems better and brighter.

- The key to peace of mind is to live in the present. You can identify what's bothering you today and plan how to work toward a resolution — one day at a time. Not all problems have solutions, but no problem or situation stays the same and most improve if you are working on them.

- Set aside daytime and early evening hours to work on or deal with problem areas, and practice turning off your mind to problems and turning it on to a relaxing routine before you go to bed. Setting a specific time to deal with problems increases overall peace of mind because you do not allow yourself to worry indiscriminately throughout the day and evening hours.

The S Word

No one is safe from the S-stress word. Regardless of lifestyle, age, or job title, you are at risk from the damaging health effects associated with stress, but there are ways to control stress and keep it from controlling you. The best defense, oddly enough, is a good offense.

Here are some ways that stress can harm your body. Like other problems mirrored by the body's largest organ — skin — stress can affect its appearance and overall healthy quality. Since stress affects body functions such as circulation and blood pressure, it in turn affects the health of major organs. Stress diminishes the body's healthy reserves and gets in the way of personal happiness and peace of mind. Not surprisingly, stress has also been linked to employment problems, family crises, divorce, accidents, illness, and just about every negative situation imaginable.

But just what is stress, where does it come from, and what are experts saying about this modern phenomenon? According to Paul J. Rosch, M.D., president of the American Institute of Stress in Yonkers, New York, "People view stress in terms of some unpleasant external threat. Often it is not the event itself that causes anxiety, but how you perceive it."

As examples of how people perceive the same situation differently, Rosch describes two different reactions to a roller-coaster ride. "Some sit with their eyes shut, white-knuckled as they clench the retaining bar. But thrill-seekers relish every steep plunge and can't wait to get on the very next ride. So it's not the roller coaster ride itself that is stressful, but what you make of it. And that's something you can frequently change or control."

For starters, here are some of the "roller coaster rides" which create stress in modern lives: bureaucratic structures where individuals feel a dwindling sense of control over their own destiny, job security, added job and home work-loads, increased job competition, fluctuating economic times, the in-creased pace of life, pressure to adapt to changing technologies, growing finan-cial demands, and information overload. All of these are very real threats to inner tranquillity — to say the least.

But once again, the situation doesn't seem to be the problem as much as one's attitude about or perception of it. Today, doctors, psychologists, businesses, and support groups are educating us about stress and helping us learn how to cope with it. We have realized that since stress is a negative factor in physical and mental health and detracts from job performance, it has absolutely no redeeming quality unless we can rechannel its energy into creativity and positive competition.

If your *reaction* to a situation rather than the situation itself is causing stress, then stress is clearly something you can control with your mind — especially if you incorporate the various techniques known to reduce stress.

Like all the quality-of-life factors we have discussed so far — from nutrition to sleep — it is essential to identify your personal stress level. How do you react to stress, what do you perceive as stressful, and where does your stress come from?

Job-related stress is a major source of the problem. Whether you are a secretary or the CEO, a desk jockey or field engineer, the pressures of mounting deadlines and increased job competition are enough to put most rational people over the edge. However, it is important to remember that when you do succumb to stress, your chances of giving your best performance are dramatically reduced. Ask any athlete or stage performer. Since they are constantly faced with handling their jobs in the highly competitive spotlight, they are no strangers to stress and its negative potential. Before a game or going on stage, athletes and performers use both physical and mental exercises to help them loosen up. They know if they are uptight, they will not perform at their highest potential.

One Thousand and One, One Thousand and Two

As you probably know, any technique or activity used to combat a stressful reaction is called stress management. The breathing technique we discussed in the chapter on eating smart is a wonderful method to use to "get a grip" on any stressful situation and help restore a sense of calm. These breathing exercises can effectively combat everything from stage fright and performance anxiety to stress-related heart palpitations and dizziness. So, begin to train yourself to be aware of increasing stressed reactions, and when you feel a stress attack coming on, start the breathing exercises. You'll calm down and be able to think more clearly about how to proceed.

Taking action against stress is important because if left unchecked, stress can be both cumulative and progressive. That means stress can snowball unless you do something about it. If you are stressed by a situation at work, that feeling can put additional pressure on other situations at work or at home. As the snowballing effect of stress grows, you may begin to feel you are on a treadmill that has run amuck. As the treadmill pace increases, your chances of getting off and walking at a normal pace seem nearly impossible.

Many people bring stress home from the job, transferring stress from one source to another, and many people have simply "burned out" early in life due to an inability to cope with the pressures. People of all ages actually become accident prone and get sick from stress, frequently experiencing dizziness, headaches, heart palpitations, indigestion, back pain, skin rashes, depression, irritability, distraction, and insomnia.

So before we yell at the kids, have a fit in traffic, kick the dog, fall down on your job performance, or get sick, let's all vow to reduce our reactions to potentially stressful situations and try not to create stress for other people. All of us know too well how difficult it is to enjoy life life when stress takes over the picture.

Here are ten tips for managing stress:

1.   Pinpoint each stress-provoking situation in your life, identifying them by where they occur: work, home, traffic, social situations, shopping, recreational activities, etc. Once you have made a written or mental list, target these situations with the stress-management techniques listed below.

2.   Identify the people and/or circumstances involved in each stress-related situation, and try to figure out how or why they trigger your stressed reaction. If you are responding to pressures they impose on you, practice being positive but assertive, and learn to say "no" and "not now" whenever necessary.

If certain people stir up uncomfortable competitive feelings, focus on setting personal goals and competing with yourself rather than on comparing yourself to others. Strive to develop your own niche which sets you apart from the crowd and allows you to excel at what you do best.

3.   Divide your list into the situations and contributing factors that you can influence or change and those you cannot. Keep in mind that even if you cannot change the stressful situation or its components, you can work on your perception of it. Remember, too, that anytime you can focus on solving a problem, you will reduce the associated stress.

4.   Improve time management and learn to "share the monkey." We've all heard the expressions "having the monkey on your back" or "putting the monkey on someone else's back." The monkey symbolizes responsibility, and people who readily assume this load come into contact with more stress than those who do not feel so responsible. Making sure the monkey gets around is one way of eliminating the amount of pressure you deal with, which in turn reduces your stress and anxiety. Here's how it works:

A co-worker comes to you with a creative suggestion or a legitimate problem that deserves further research or action. Instead of offering to look into the matter or promising to get back in touch, try delegating to the creative thinker who brought you the idea or problem in the first place. Downloading and sharing responsibility helps reduce your stress and encourages a team approach, which is good for any group of people. Sharing the monkey relieves pressures and demands on your time and allows co-workers to feel involved in the progress of the organization. You can also use this approach with family members and friends.

5.   When there are heavy demands on your time, stress runs high. It is absolutely necessary to make time for yourself to do something you enjoy, that gets your mind completely off your routine. This quality time is like the release valve on a pressure cooker that provides an escape for steam. If you keep saying that you do not have time for yourself and cannot take time away from your job or responsibilities, one day you really may not have time . . . period.

6.   Healthy exercise (especially aerobics) and balanced nutrition, as well as routine and consistent sleep, are major antistress factors. These are the components which enable you to perform at your potential and help you think and react clearly, calmly, and rationally when you are under stress.

7.   Typically the people most susceptible to stress and related illnesses and problems are those known as Type A behavior or perfectionists. They are obsessively concerned with details and feel they have to be involved in order to get the job done right.

If you are one of these people, work on how you talk to yourself. Try removing "should" from your vocabulary, eliminating any thought that perfection exists anywhere, and dismiss any thought that your way is the only "right" way to do things.

8. If you are prone to feeling anxious or nervous and are susceptible to stress, limit caffeine, which can stimulate such reactions. Many people drink coffee, tea, and soft drinks containing caffeine throughout the day. More than 250 to 300 mg of caffeine a day (approximately 2 to 4 cups of coffee) and over-the-counter medications containing caffeine can contribute to jittery, irritable reactions.

9. If you are the quiet type who feels a lot of stress but keeps it all inside, it is very important to find ways in which you can release your pent-up feelings and frustrations. Talking to someone who will be supportive helps, and learning to become comfortable expressing your feelings is actually good for your health. Take advantage of your quiet reputation. When people who are generally quiet and reserved speak up, others tend to take them very seriously and listen to what they have to say.

10. There are limits to what stress management can do to help you. If your anxiety or fears are prolonged or severe, please get help from your physician or a referral to someone who specializes in dealing with stress.

Chill Out, As They Say

Whatever you do, take a break from stress. In the scope of things, life is so very short and every single day is precious. Stress harms your health and happiness, your job performance, and your relationships, but coping with stress is a matter of education and action. There is no mystery surrounding it. Like a few other negatives we will discuss in this chapter, stress is a very controllable, avoidable factor in our lives. Once you realize that stress is a cunning and powerful enemy, an opponent that manipulates your mind and depletes your powers, it is easy to close the door in its face.

Smoking and Second-Hand Smoke

Smoking and second-hand smoke are tremendous threats to the lives of smokers and nonsmokers alike. Even if you do not smoke or quit years ago, please read on because we all know people who continue to smoke despite constant warnings. These smokers are harming our health by polluting the air we breathe and doing incredible damage to their own health in the process. People who continue to smoke turn those of us who do not smoke into involuntary smokers. There's a big

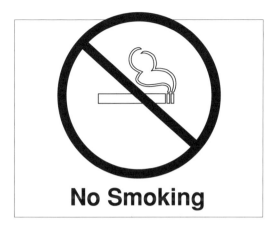

No Smoking

health risk associated with involuntary smoking, and those of us who are victims of second-hand smoke need to understand the specific health problems we face. The information in this section should be considered ammunition for the cause.

Here are some important Did-You-Know Facts from the American Cancer Society:

Secondary Smoke

• If you have ever breathed the smoke that curls up from the tip of someone's cigarette or the smoke exhaled by a smoker, then you have breathed most of the same harmful, cancer-causing parts of smoke inhaled by smokers. That actually makes you an involuntary smoker and puts you at a greatly disadvantaged health risk.

• The Environmental Protection Agency (EPA) estimates that 3,700 lung-cancer deaths annually — nearly 3 percent of the annual lung-cancer death toll — have been caused by involuntary smoking.

• Involuntary smoking causes lung cancer and heart disease, aggravates asthmatic conditions, and impairs blood circulation.

• Studies show that people who live with smokers are especially at risk. Nonsmokers married to habitual smokers were found to have a two to three times greater risk of lung cancer compared with those married to nonsmokers.

• An American Cancer Society study found that nonsmokers exposed to twenty or more cigarettes a day at home had twice the risk of developing lung cancer than people exposed to fewer cigarettes.

• People who are exposed to smokers in the workplace are also at risk. Even if you do not sit next to or near a smoker, the smoky air circulates through the air.

• Children who are exposed to second-hand smoke have a greater chance of developing colds, bronchitis, pneumonia (especially during the first two years of life), chronic coughs, ear infections, and reduced lung function.

Smoking Spells Death and Disease

• Because lung cancer is difficult to detect early, it is very difficult to treat successfully. It is often fatal. If no one smoked cigarettes, 83 percent of lung cancer would eventually disappear.

• Cigarette smoking tells a very ugly story — inside and out. Its effects are devastating to the skin, lungs, and other organs of the body.

• Smokers have a higher rate of death than nonsmokers: one-half pack a day causes a 30 percent higher rate; one to two packs, 100 percent higher; over two packs, 140 percent higher.

• The lung-cancer death rate for women has risen 425 percent over the thirty years since women started smoking as much as men.

Women and Smoking

• Pregnant women who smoke are smoking for two. Their babies have decreased birth weights and have more chance of being stillborn or dying within the first month. The nicotine, carbon monoxide, and dangerous chemicals in smoke enter the mother's bloodstream and pass into the baby's body.

• When women combine smoking with oral contraception, they are ten times more likely to suffer a heart attack than nonsmoking women who do not take birth control pills. They have an increased risk of stroke and blood clots in the legs. Older female smokers have an increased risk of osteoporosis, and all women smokers increase their risk of getting cancer of the uterine cervix.

• Despite massive educational campaigns, the progress women are making in antismoking efforts doesn't look good. Between 1965 and 1987, male smoking rates decreased by more than 18 percent, but female smoking rates fell by only about 5 percent. Do you think those cigarette ads, disguised in pro-feminist messages claiming "You've come a long way, baby," tell the real story?

• Lung and breast cancer are the two leading cancers which cause death in women today. The increased incident of both is directly linked to smoking.

Teenagers Who Smoke

• It is estimated that more than 3,000 U.S. teenagers start smoking every day — over 1 million each year. Current statistics predict that if these young smokers grow up to smoke at current adult rates, at least 5 million of them will die of smoking-related diseases.

• A survey of high school seniors showed that girls smoke more than boys, and that college-bound students smoke less than students without higher education plans.

• The highest rates of smokeless tobacco use (chewing tobacco and snuff) are found among young males. Approximately 1.7 million boys between the ages of 12 and 17 have used some form of smokeless tobacco. Smokeless tobacco is heavily linked to cancer of the mouth, tooth loss, and gum damage.

The Economics of Smoking

The big question is why smoking has not been banned all together — especially in view of the strong position Congress, the Environmental Protection Agency, and the Food and Drug Administration take toward any product or device which is harmful or hazardous to our health. The answer, no doubt, is economics — or is it politics?

The tobacco industry is one of the most profitable businesses in this country and one of the most powerful lobbying groups in Washington, but ironically, the actual costs of smoking are far higher than the tremendous income generated by cigarette sales.

According to information from the American Cancer Society, in 1985, cigarette sales contributed approximately $32 billion to the American economy. Of this, approximately $8.9 billion went to federal, state, and local taxes, and more than $3 billion went to companies' profits. However, the Office of Technology Assessment has estimated that health-care costs — including Medicare and Medicaid — for treating smoking-related diseases amounted to approximately $22 billion during the same year. The cost of lost earnings from early death and disease due to smoking was about $43 billion. The yearly total amounted to approximately $65 billion in financial costs and immeasurable pain, suffering, and loss experienced by those people who were crippled or killed by cigarettes — not to mention the devastating grief suffered by their families. With our current knowledge of the harmful effects and financial losses caused by cigarettes, it is difficult to imagine how tobacco is still legal in this country, especially in view of the economic arguments the industry uses to justify its existence.

What Can Be Done?

Like all other health matters, education is linked to progress. Both the private and public sectors have taken actions which have led to a decrease in the number of smoking-related deaths and illnesses in this country. Warning labels appear on all packaging. Advertising on radio and television has been banned. A majority of states have voted to limit minors' access to tobacco products. Many work environments and public places have become smoke free, and Congress has banned smoking on domestic airplane flights.

Smoking is a matter of addiction, and millions of smokers struggle with their addictions. For those who breathe their smoke second hand, the risk of dying from cancers caused by passive smoking is more than three times greater than the risk of dying from cancers caused by all other air pollutants. Statistics show that of 100 regular smokers in the United States, 1 will be murdered, 2 will die in traffic accidents, and 25 will die from tobacco use.

Cigarette smoking kills 390,000 Americans each year — the same number of people who would die if three jumbo jets crashed with no survivors every day for one year. In all, smoking is responsible for one in six deaths in the United States and is the single most preventable cause of death in our society. This is a massive health hazard to both smokers and second-hand smokers. In essence, smoking concerns every one of us in one way or another.

There are a variety of organizations and support groups that provide services, information, and help. To get help or request further information — even if you've quit smoking and started back — contact these organizations:

American Cancer Society
1599 Clifton Road, N.E.
Atlanta, GA 30329
(800) ACS-2345

National Cancer Institute
9000 Rockville Pike
Bldg. 31, Room 4A-18
Bethesda, MD 20892
(800) 4-CANCER

American Heart Association National
    Center
7320 Greenville Avenue
Dallas, TX 75231
(214) 750-5300

Office on Smoking and Health
Centers for Disease Control
5600 Fishers Lane

Park Building, Room 1-16
Rockville, MD 20857
(301) 443-5287

American Lung Association
1740 Broadway
New York, NY 10019-4374
(212) 315-8700

Just remember . . . smoking never offers a room with a view of a good and healthy life.

Here's to Your Health

Like smoking, drinking alcoholic beverages is often glamorized and associated with sophisticated people enjoying "the good life." But unlike smoking, which has no redeeming qualities, alcoholic beverages — from the finest wines to aged liquors and the most refreshing beers — are fine in moderation. The only problems come with excess or misuse.

Drinking too much alcohol or drinking at the wrong times can cause deterioration in both the body and mind. For example, alcohol robs the body of certain vitamins and nutrients — especially vitamin B, which alcohol borrows from the body's reserves to be metabolized. Vitamin B has been called the brain vitamin because it is associated with memory and brain function. For the sake of sheer brain power, it is very important to be sure the body does not get depleted of this valuable resource.

But that's not all. Deficiencies of

vitamin B also cause an inability to concentrate, insomnia, and lack of initiative. Studies show that alcohol-induced memory loss can increase with age. Loss of vitamin B is not only associated with drinking alcoholic beverages but also smoking and taking certain drugs such as tranquilizers, barbiturates, diuretics, beta blockers, and anti-inflammatory medications.

Some people mistakenly think that it is possible to make up for vitamin B loss by eating foods high in the vitamin or by taking vitamin B supplements. Replacing lost nutrients and rebuilding the body's reserves may help in some ways, but nothing helps the damage done to your memory which is caused by drinking too much, smoking cigarettes, or taking certain drugs. As a matter of fact, memory loss can remain after the self-destructive behavior has stopped.

Alcohol and certain foods high in sugar content such as candy have much in common. Both are high in calories that are of little or no use to the body, and both deplete the body of vitamin B. For anyone concerned with reducing or maintaining weight and overall body-fat levels, alcoholic drinks can be an unneeded calorie source. The average alcoholic drink contains between 150 and 300 calories. When these calories are combined with regular foods, it doesn't take many drinks for the total daily calorie count to go sky high.

Alcohol also depletes the body of fluids because it increases urination. Never drink alcoholic drinks shortly before, during, or right after exercise.

Many people combine physical activities with beverages such as beer, or they drink beer and other alcoholic drinks when they are outdoors basking in the sun. This is not a very smart idea because alcohol increases the loss of body fluids and results in dehydration. Plus, basking in the sun destroys your skin. You will regret the tan that you think makes you look so good today (a subject to be discussed in detail later).

There is an old Chinese proverb that says, "Good sense is the master of human life." When it comes to drinking alcohol, this is the best advice; there is nothing wrong with having one to two drinks in an evening, but any more than two ounces of alcohol a day crosses the line between pleasurable relaxation and bodily abuse.

Mental Powers

As far as humorous sayings go, the quip "Of all the things I've lost, I miss my mind the most" is most appropriate here. Loss of mental power is sometimes mistaken for a part of the natural aging process, but in fact, the mind can stay bright and clear as we age. We can actually grow smarter as we gather knowledge and learn from cumulative experiences.

Yes, senility happens, but it is not the norm. The brain can keep working and functioning properly for a very long and lucid lifetime. Aging does not have to mean mental deterioration. However, the keys to mental power are taking care of ourselves — both body and mind — and maintaining a mentally active, challenging, and stimulating life.

Let's take a good look at the way in which the brain ages. As we grow older, there is a gradual slowdown in our ability to learn and solve problems, but research shows that as long as there is no accident, disease, or extreme stress, the brain does not become worn out with age. There is, however, some degree of progressive memory loss — especially in short-term memory.

There are two kinds of memory. Short-term memory refers to those things you remember and recall quickly such as the name of a person you hear upon being introduced. You remember the name a few minutes later and recall it in conversation. Long-term memory refers to those things you remember from the past, such as the address of the house where you grew up over thirty years ago. Of the two kinds of memory, long-term memory is generally the stronger. This explains why your grandmother could relate a detailed story from her childhood but could not remember where she put her purse. The difference is that long-term memories usually have been repeated and reinforced, but short-term memories deal with new information that requires spontaneous recall.

As aging occurs and the brain gradually slows down, there are — as you know — many older people who remain very bright, focused, and alert. This is one of the major ways in which younger people make comparisons between their elders. How many times have you heard someone say, "He's in his eighties, but he doesn't miss a beat." The biggest difference seems to be that although the aging brain may slow down, older people who are mentally active and stimulated naturally compensate for this decrease with knowledge, experience, and careful persistence.

Also, scientists are dispelling the idea that the brain is one of the few organs of the body that cannot repair itself. As a matter of fact, new research indicates that the brain makes up for any lost cells by making new cell connections, that parts of the brain do not lose cells at all, and that certain parts of the brain continue to grow — even well into old age.

In a widely cited study Robert L. Kahn, Ph.D., of the University of Chicago concluded that many older people complained of having poor memory, but their complaint did not jibe with their performance on memory tests. This evidence points to the fact that people fear aging and memory loss and become distrustful of their own mental powers, and that many older people who are actually suffering from depression confuse those symptoms with poor memory.

This kind of emotional depression is associated with illness, bereavement, loneliness, lack of stimulating activity, and economic problems — all of which can be common to older people at one time or another. Two aspects of depression work in tandem in a negative way to prolong both the blue feelings and perceived memory loss. When you are feeling low, your memory doesn't work as well — which makes you feel even worse and makes your memory work even less. This can be a vicious circle until steps are taken in the right direction to improve the problem.

First of all, in order to maximize your memory and your mental powers, you must exercise your mind in order to keep it strong and fit, just as you exercise your body for the same reasons. People who are deprived of an active, stimulating environment typically grow dull and unhappy, just as people who have no physical activity grow fat and lazy. Research shows that people who engage in tasks and activities which require regular concentration and problem-solving skills maintain their mental abilities better and are mentally sharper longer than those who do not.

And if short-term memory is a problem — at any age — try creating memory quizzes that you can give yourself. For example, read a list of 25 words and then try to write down all the words you can remember. The more you practice this quiz, the better your short-term memory will get. Also use memory techniques such as constructing mental images of lists of words you want to remember. Try practicing this technique on your daily "to-do" list or grocery list. The more you practice, the better you'll get at visualizing and remembering. You can also use this visual image technique to improve your ability to remember names. When you first meet someone, immediately connect a strong visual image with the person's name. For example, you meet a Mr. Adams. Think of any distinct and memorable advertisement that sticks in your mind. Picture Mr. Adams in that ad. The next time you see Mr. Adams, you will probably recall the mental image of a man in an ad—thus the connection—ad and Adams. Such mental games may sound silly, but they work. As a matter of fact, the more outrageous and vivid your images are, the better your chance of making a memory connection.

Use It or Lose It

People like to be mentally challenged — unless they have gotten lazy from a lack of stimulation — in which case they tend to forget how fulfilling mental challenges can really be. But the mind, like the body, is subject to another adage: "Use it or lose it."

The more you use your brain, the more stimulated it becomes. The more mentally active you are, the clearer and more alert the memory. There is no doubt that people who are involved in challenging, creative activities have greater mental powers, and people who get plenty of physical exercise have healthier bodies.

We've all heard the term "brain food" before, and there's a lot of truth there. In order to maximize mental power and enhance memory, there are certain foods which are good to eat. In a study conducted under the auspices of the National Institute of Mental Health, a vitamin-like substance called choline has been closely linked to efficient brain function and memory enhancement.

This study involved normal, healthy volunteers who took one ten-gram dose of choline and were able to memorize a sequence of unrelated words more quickly than normal. The study also showed that the people whose memories were the poorest were those whose memories were helped the most by taking the choline. (Foods which are good sources of choline include soybean, beef liver, eggs, and fish.)

As we discussed in the preceding section on alcohol, deficiency of vitamin B is also linked to brain disturbances and memory loss. Thiamine (vitamin B-1) deficiency is sometimes mistaken for senility and is a contributing cause of insomnia and lethargy. These deficiencies can be improved by eating foods that are good sources of vitamin B nutrients, such as brewer's yeast, beef liver, sunflower seeds, dried soybeans, kidney beans, and other beans which contain thiamine.

Everything you do to keep yourself healthy and fit is good for each organ of the body, including the brain, but it is a good idea to find out exactly what the brain thrives on. Avoiding vitamin B deficiencies, steering clear of excessive use of alcohol and drugs which rob the body of vitamin B, and getting plenty of sleep and stress-free relaxation are good starts. However, it is necessary to exercise the mind in order to prolong and maintain mental fitness throughout all the days of your life.

Can Older Be Better?

As long as good health prevails, midlife represents the most stable and dependable years for the majority of people. At midlife, we are better able to handle whatever changes life brings our way. Over the years we have accumulated more skills and knowledge and are better able to manage ourselves than ever before. For many, midlife brings an awareness of the finite quality of life, and we respond by recognizing that every day of our lives counts and by trying to make the most of life.

Midlife is a thoughtful time in our lives. It brings us to a point where we see many of our goals becoming reality, where what we planned and worked for so hard begins to be less of a burden and more of a pleasure. At the same time, many people entering midlife are still reaching toward their goals, expanding horizons, and accepting challenges beyond their original expectations. Fortunately, midlife gives us the leading edge of experience. We are old enough to do anything and young enough to do anything.

There is no reason to dread growing older — especially today when there are so many wonderful opportunities and such a wealth of knowledge about how to stay young and look and feel your best. And there is no doubt that older can be better, especially for positive thinkers and active people.

When you hear someone fantasize about returning to a younger day, he or she will invariably add, "But only if I could know what I know now." This statement is a clear indication of our values — that the experience and knowledge we have earned throughout our lives are highly regarded assets and that we wouldn't trade them . . . even for the promise of youth.

Formula for a Long and Happy Life

If we combine our basic knowledge of anti-aging, health, and fitness with sound nutrition and the components for personal happiness, here's how it all comes together.

1. Eat breakfast to get a good start for the day. Eat balanced meals and limit animal fats by eating moderate portions of meat, eggs, poultry, and fish. Include lots of fruits and vegetables. Limit amounts of fat, oil, and sugar, and avoid in-between-meal snacks. Adults: Get plenty of complex carbohydrates.

2. Eat whole-grain products every day.

3. Drink lots of water (8 glasses) per day. (Do not count coffee, tea, juice, or sodas, and keep them to a minimum.)

4. Drink only moderate amounts of alcoholic beverages, if any.

5. Do not smoke or use any tobacco products.

6. Exercise at least three to five times a week to burn fat and build muscle. (Consult your doctor first.)

7. Maintain a consistent body weight and monitor percentage of body fat according to healthy levels set by your physician.

8. Sleep seven to eight hours per night regularly.

9. Reduce and manage stress, and learn to relax.

10. Build satisfying personal relationships and open communications.

11. Maintain a feeling of control over your life and pursue both personal interests and new opportunities.

12. Create a stimulating environment that is both mentally challenging and personally enjoyable.

LOOKING GOOD OUTSIDE, FEELING GOOD INSIDE

Dermatology and cosmetic surgery will probably be around until such time as they repeal the law of gravity.
—Drs. Elson and Hartley

Each of us is concerned about how we look and about how our appearance will change over the years. These concerns are natural and actually very good for us, because making the most of appearance, preventing premature aging, and maximizing health simply mean we are taking care of ourselves. Making sure we look as good on the outside as we feel on the inside is part of being the best we can be.

The good news is that dermatology and cosmetic surgery offer increasing opportunities to protect against the skin's aging process, protect the skin from environmental damage, improve physical defects, and enhance physical features. In the last decade alone, many new medical advances and scientific developments have offered tremendous self-improvement options in both cosmetic surgery and nonsurgical procedures. We have never had such a great opportunity to look good before. So here's your chance to learn all about those opportunities and to discover the incredible connection between looking good on the outside and on the inside.

Skin Care and Cosmetics: An Ancient Art

Before discussing the sophisticated skin-care opportunities of our day, let's get a bit of historical perspective. Skin care dates back to the ancient Egyptians. They created elaborate systems for bathing and after bathing, lubricated their skin with oils, lotions, and ointments. Cleopatra, queen of Egypt (51 B.C.), is said to have lavished cosmetics and fragrances on her body, face, hair, and nails. The early Hebrews were also highly conscious of health and cleanliness, and they were known for their beautiful skin and hair. The Hebrews learned to manufacture many preparations for the skin, hair, nails, and teeth, and some of the Bible's earliest books record their use of fragrances to anoint the heads of their honored guests.

The Greeks had what is referred to as the most culturally advanced civilization when it reached its heights in the years 460 to 146 B.C. Displaying great interest in the beauty of the skin, they made lavish use of cosmetic products for both personal and medicinal purposes. Greek women used facial preparations to improve the quality of their skin and enhance their appearances — white lead to even out the tone of their complexions, kohl to darken their eyes, and vermilion (a brilliant red pigment powder) to color their lips. Both Greek men and women understood the importance of bathing and cleansing the skin, as well as lubricating the skin's surface to keep it soft and supple.

The ancient Romans borrowed many skin-care and cosmetic practices from the Greeks and developed many more of their own. They were devoted users of fragrances and cosmetic preparations. In about 454 B.C., the practice of shaving the face became popular for men, and a clean-shaven face became the modern style. Roman women used facial cleansing preparations made from milk and bread and sometimes fine wine and others made from corn, flour, and milk mixed with fresh butter. They made cosmetic mixtures from chalk and white lead which they dusted on their faces to smooth their complexions, reddened their lips with vegetable dyes, and darkened their eyelids and eyebrows with makeup made from kohl. The Romans are famous for their elaborate public buildings with separate baths for men and women. After the bathing ritual, they used rich oils and lotions to keep the skin soft and attractive.

Throughout history the Orientals have advanced many skin-care practices, as have the Africans, who are known for developing medicinal and grooming preparations from substances found in their own environments. Regardless of culture, from the earliest time to the present day, people have been concerned with preserving and improving the quality of their skin because healthy skin has long been recognized as vital to an attractive appearance and good health. In fact, in most cultures the science of cosmetology and medicine have been closely linked throughout the ages.

Self-Image

Your self-image is a composite of all the mental pictures you have of yourself. It is a combination of all you have heard about yourself from others and what you have told yourself. Your self-image is a record of past experiences — from the reinforcement you have received in your family, with friends, and at the workplace.

Can you summarize your self-image? Just take a sheet of paper and start brainstorming all the adjectives that best describe you. It is important to be as objective as possible. Once you get that part of your brain which controls descriptive adjectives warmed up, match your adjectives to these self-image categories. Write a word or two beside each one.

1. facial appearance
2. quality of skin
3. hair
4. body size and shape
5. weight
6. fitness

After you have described yourself in each of these categories, go back and reread what you wrote. How many words were positive? How many were negative? Put a plus sign (+) by the positives and a negative sign (−) by the negatives.

No one really needs to tell you how to score this exercise. The objective here is simply to get you to see in black-and-white terms how you judge your appearance and to sort out the positives from the negatives. The beauty of this exercise is that those categories which include positive descriptions can even get stronger and last longer. And a negative aspect doesn't have to last forever.

This book deals primarily with what makes you feel good on the inside and look good on the outside. We do not talk about personal ability, achievement, and happiness, but we'll be willing to wager that if you get all the other categories in this exercise up to a positive level, then ability, achievement, and happiness won't be far behind.

Why are we so sure? Because the way you look and feel about yourself influences everything.

Appearance Counts

Remember, this book is not about beauty or trying to reach an ideal image. It's about self-esteem and all the components that can improve self-esteem. Self-esteem is greatly influenced by appearance, and it affects much more

than just how we feel about ourselves. The perception we have of how other people feel about us in large part determines how we present ourselves and how we interact with others.

Appearance influences everything from our social lives to our professional careers. The media has even gone so far as to refer to cosmetic surgery as "success surgery" and "psychological surgery" because of the profound effect positive change has on people's lives. People notice when you make improvements, and as you look better, positive energy abounds. Friends and co-workers always notice when you wear new clothes, change your hair style or hair color, lose weight, and get in shape. They tell you when you look tired and worried, rested and relaxed. Not only are we interested in our own appearances, we are very aware of the appearance of those around us. It's human nature.

Everyone notices, and everyone has an opinion. People may not have noticed you for months, but when you make a change in your appearance, everyone perks up. We like to see others improve themselves. We encourage each other to do so. Of course, not everyone's opinion will be the same, and that's why the decisions you make about your appearance are, most importantly, up to you.

Bob Barker, the Emmy award–winning television host of "The Price Is Right," who has twice been named to the *Guinness Book of World Records* as television's "most durable performer," knows just how much appearance

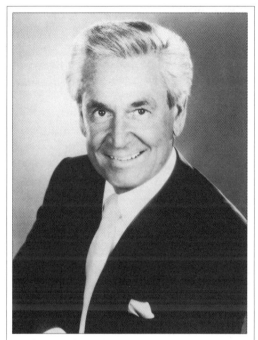

TV host Bob Barker

in advance before vacation that audiences never realized I was gone. When I returned, we picked up and 'The Price Is Right' never missed a day on television. On Tuesday, my hair was dark. On Wednesday, my hair was completely gray. The audience gasped when they saw me. I had so many supportive letters, and the overall response was 99.9 percent positive. One man wrote to say he liked my new look, but he hoped I was feeling okay because somewhere between Tuesday and Wednesday, I must have had one heck of a night."

Skin: The Great Cover Up

Like hair, skin is readily noticeable, and people pay attention to it. Skin plays an important role in personal appearance because it covers the entire body. At one time or another, every area of skin shows.

Skin has been called the wrapping of the human package because it holds the entire body together. It is usually the first thing people notice when they look at each other's faces and bodies. Skin is a very prominent part of the impression you make and the image you have of yourself.

Sometimes we take normal, healthy skin for granted, but it requires special attention to stay that way. Caring for your skin is an essential health issue; throughout life, skin is subject to

counts. His television show and numerous personal appearances put him in front of the public every day. Although he is more mature than when he began his successful career years ago, he is just as attractive and fun loving today as he was at any other stage of his life.

"A positive appearance is very valuable in any walk of life," Barker said, "because people really do notice how you look. For years, I tinted my hair to cover the gray, and then I decided to stop. I went on vacation and decided to let my hair go *au naturel*. By the end of the trip, I was completely gray. When I returned to the show, my producer, Bud Grant, liked my new look so well that I decided to let the gray alone. The funny part was that I had taped enough shows problems that range from complexion irregularities to wrinkles and creases, from age spots to potentially life-threatening premalignant and malignant lesions. As a matter of fact, in a 1971–74 Health and Nutritional Examination survey conducted by the U.S. Census Bureau, two-thirds of a representative sampling of adults over seventy years of age had skin conditions considered serious enough to warrant medical attention.

The point is, people of all ages have skin problems which can become bigger problems down the road if they aren't treated. Older people do not acquire skin problems overnight or as soon as they reach a certain age. Problems affecting the skin usually occur very gradually over time, and many of them are preventable or treatable. Skin care begins in infancy and continues throughout life, so there is never a good time to take your skin for granted or ignore its special needs.

This giant, wonderful organ is known to be the most dependable and potentially long-lasting organ of the body in maintaining its primary function of protecting the body from physical and chemical assaults. The moral to any skin story is that if you care for your skin, it can serve and support you very well for many years, but when things go wrong with your skin, the results can be embarrassing, uncomfortable, painful, and threatening to your health.

If you feel people are paying atten-tion to detracting physical characteristics such as acne scars, wrinkles, crow's feet, and sagging skin, it affects your self-esteem and how you interact with others. Some of the most ingrained self-esteem problems we see are direct results of unattractive skin conditions — most commonly acne, acne scars, and wrinkles.

As already mentioned, our perception of how others see us and how they interact with us influences both our opinion of ourselves and our behavior toward others. If you are self-conscious about perceived flaws or embarrassed about certain physical features, these feelings affect all other feelings. The following real stories illustrate just how influential appearance can be on both personality and self-esteem.

Courtney (Age 16)

One of our patients is an attractive sixteen-year-old girl who suffers from acne, which is particularly severe on her cheeks and forehead. Although she has a nice figure, pretty facial features, and many other positive attributes, she has grown her hair long and wears it straight down, covering her forehead and as much of her cheeks as possible. When she looks up from out of all this hair covering her face, all you can see are eyes, nose, and mouth. No amount of pleading from her very supportive parents has altered her hair style.

Her parents say that ever since the acne problem became acute, they have noticed that she has become much more withdrawn, spending most of her time away from school alone in her room. She talks on the phone to friends but does not go out as much as she used to.

Her mother remarked, "Before this year, I couldn't keep Courtney home. Now, I can't get her to go out with her friends. It's as if her personality has changed — almost overnight."

Stephen (Age 33)

Another patient who came to us for treatment of acne scarring was a young man in his early thirties who was tall and well built and had classically handsome facial features. Unfortunately, a severe case of teenage acne had left deep scars on both cheeks, and the trauma of the acne left his complexion very red and ruddy looking, as it often does.

This young man was extremely shy. It was difficult for him to hold eye contact during conversation, and he became very nervous when the nurses in the office asked him questions requiring direct answers. He was self-conscious and insecure. His body language gave away his emotions. It was like reading an open book.

We saw him over the course of the next several weeks, treating him with dermabrasion to smooth and even out the skin's texture and with collagen-replacement therapy to fill in the scarred areas. As his complexion improved and the scars became less noticeable, this young man became a different person. The progress we were making with his skin was mirrored by the way his personality changed.

He became very friendly and so much more open and outgoing. He readily looked us straight in the eye during conversation, and his sense of humor emerged as he joked with the nurses in the office. It sounds amazing, but once we freed this young man from his problem, he became the person he really was all the while.

On return visits to the office, we all noticed how attractively dressed he was and how happy he seemed. One day, he was in an especially good mood and announced to us that he became engaged to a young woman he had met just six months ago. All of us in the office couldn't help but feel proud and happy for him. We also felt good about our work because the best part of what we do is evident when we have a chance to see someone like Stephen metamorphosing before our very eyes. The opportunity to see someone come out of a shell and begin to realize his potential is terrific.

Alexis (Age 48)

For the last several years, we treated Alexis with injectable collagen to improve scars she had on her face from acne. She had gone through the pain of adolescent acne which continued as adult acne, and it was only after the birth of her children that the problem began to subside.

She also has heavy fold lines below the cheeks just above the corners of her mouth. These kinds of folds are very common and are determined by heredity, although they tend to become more noticeable with age and as gravity works on the skin. We used collagen to build-up these fold lines in her skin and have improved her facial contour as a result.

Alexis is a very upbeat person,

self-confident and in tune with her appearance. She is a very attractive woman, but until now she said she felt helpless to do anything about the scars on her cheeks. She says that although she tried to ignore them by focusing on other good features, she never got over wanting the scars to go away.

Alexis comes to the office every five or six months to have collagen treatments, and about a year ago, she had a facelift and eyelid surgery which her friends told her made her look 15 years younger. She is very pleased with her improvements overall, but she says that making the scars less noticeable was the biggest psychological lift of all.

Learning to Like Yourself

Many counselors and therapists spend years trying to teach people how to like themselves, how to get over and grow beyond the burden of low self-esteem. They understand the widespread negative effect it has on people's lives.

Research shows that people who feel good about themselves actually tend to live longer, happier lives. So, feeling good about the way you look is a very valid reason for analyzing yourself and learning about self-improvement options. The information in this chapter will help you learn more about yourself and about the options which can enhance your appearance and health. We will give you some basic background on how skin works, what causes skin to age, and how to keep skin healthy. We will provide an overview of skin care, skin-treatment options, and medical options and surgical procedures which can improve skin problems and physical features. Overall, we continue to blend educational information with encouraging words about self-improvement because we can all benefit from positive thinking and motivation where appearance and health are concerned.

There is no reason for anyone in this modern age to suffer from any physical feature or condition which they consider unattractive or undesirable. If there is a prevention or treatment for something that bothers you, you should examine all the options. From acne to aging, creases to wrinkles, scars to pox marks, hair problems to out-of-proportion facial or body features — these and many other conditions can be changed, improved, and enhanced.

Sore Spots in Our Self-Esteem

When people are concerned about physical characteristics or features, it is difficult for them to see past what they perceive sets them apart in a negative way. Every time they look in the mirror or at a photograph — every day of their lives — they are painfully aware of a sore spot in their self-esteem. Even though they may spend money to buy good-looking clothes, create attractive hair styles, and learn to apply cosmetics, there is little if anything that makes them forget the physical characteristic they do not like or are embarrassed about. The miracles of cosmetic dermatology and cosmetic plastic surgery have enhanced many lives by unlocking positive self-esteem.

As psychologist, author, and lecturer Perry W. Buffington, Ph.D., explains, "In counseling men and women of all ages, I discovered that cosmetic surgery has accomplished many positive therapeutic results which years of psychotherapy failed to provide. When people are dissatisfied with their appearances and feel helpless to change, it is very difficult for psychotherapy to build self-esteem regarding appearance. Self-esteem and self-acceptance are key to personal beauty — inside and out."

When you consider how the histories of dermatology and plastic surgery evolved beyond the areas of critical response, it is interesting to note that we soon began to treat the psyche as well as the physique. Throughout history, as soon as we made progress in preventing fatal diseases and achieved advances in treating critical injuries, we turned to learning more about diseases, deformities, defects, and problems that were not so much life threatening as emotionally destructive.

Marion Sulzberger was acutely aware of how self-esteem affected the human psyche. He parleyed his great intellect and energy into becoming one of the foremost dermatologists who ever lived, serving as chairman of the department of dermatology at New York University and later on the faculty of the University of California at San Francisco.

The story of how he initially decided to go into the field of dermatology is very touching. His sister, Dulcie, had a significant acne problem as a teenager growing up in Switzerland in the early 1900s. Her problem was so severe at one point that she became totally despondent and was unable to eat or get out of bed for a long time. When all available treatments did not cure her acne, she actually attempted suicide. Fortunately, the gun she held in her hand did not fire. Her brother was very sensitive to suffering of any type, and he was so moved by his sister's case and so distraught by the traumatic effect of her skin disease and its permanent scarring of her skin as well as her emotions that he began his lifelong dedication to the treatment of acne and other skin diseases.

There is a great deal more to how the world sees you than what is on the surface, but it is also very true that scars, lines, and imperfections of the skin are more than skin deep. There are scars of the psyche as well as scars of the skin, and while most people's faces may not be their fortunes, your face influences your every move and affects almost every thought you have. That is why it is so important to put your best face forward, to be comfortable with how you look, and to feel good about yourself.

The Patience Factor

You have taken the first steps by reading this book and beginning to act on constructive self-improvement ideas that are good for you. Once you really get started on any self-improvement goal, the next step is to develop the patience it will take to see you through to progress and results. One of the shortcomings people have is that they do not give a program enough time to work before they change it and head off in another direction. We see this "restless resolve" over and over again. People want to make positive changes, but they start and stop, start and stop, start and stop, which is very frustrating, expensive, and self-defeating.

Take skin-care programs, for example. Results of skin care take time and consistency, but while many of us make a commitment to get involved in skin care, go out and spend money buying what we think is necessary to improve our skin, before long we lose interest and give up — only to renew our commitment by purchasing other products later on. How many neat little bottles and jars do you have in your collection?

If impatience is not a problem in your skin care program, how about in your diet or work-out routine? How many times have you bought new sports shoes or equipment, joined health clubs, bought exercise equipment, and embarked — with new resolve — to shape up? The point is, we seem to be longer on resolution than on the patience needed to focus and fulfill our good intentions, and many people confuse starting and stopping and investing money with making at least some degree of progress. This is not valid.

In addition to the desire to change or improve your appearance and making the commitment to do so, progress and results require patience. There are no overnight success stories. Just as you must fuel your ideas with actions, so you must fund your goals with the time it takes to get realistic results.

Let's say, for example, that you want to improve your appearance and decide to investigate cosmetic dermatology or cosmetic surgery. You must patiently approach the educational process involved in learning what procedure is the right one for you and who is the right doctor to perform the procedure. You'll need to be patient during the actual procedure, which may take more than one visit to the doctor's office or surgicenter, and you'll need patience during the healing and recovery process which follows.

Mother Nature is very patient in how she changes our faces and bodies. Gradually, over time the everyday stress of muscles working and gravity pulling take their toll on your skin. In order to counteract the forces of nature and the natural aging process, you must respond with the same simple, patient approach that nature herself takes. Make a minimum number of corrective changes at a time so as not to become overwhelmed, and aim your future efforts at preventive measures rather than at correcting mistakes. Unfortunately, there are no miracle creams — just simple preventive steps and corrective measures which can, if properly performed, make the most of your skin and your good looks for many years.

Stow-Away Stigmas

A discussion about improving appearance is a good place to review your attitudes and ideas about self-improvement. The experiences you have had over the course of your lifetime influence how you think and act today. What you have been told — especially by people who were very opinionated or who played key roles in your life — makes a lasting impression. Many adults in this world make decisions and take action based on impressions and prejudices which were formed long ago. When is the last time you really reviewed how you make decisions about yourself?

Do you make your own decisions? Do you have an open mind about new opportunities? Do you think you look attractive or unattractive based on how someone else makes you feel? Do you hide from or avoid taking care of yourself? Do you not take the time for yourself because you are so busy with work or taking care of other people? Do your responses involve preconceived notions, or do you take a defensive position without knowing all the facts? Are you conditioned to rationalize your thoughts or, in other words, tell yourself

what you need to hear? When is the last time you told yourself the truth?

Let's look at something so simple as the way in which you approach skin care. You learned very early in life about the importance of cleansing your skin because someone was probably always reminding you to wash your face and hands. But as adults, many people still harbor a dislike for washing their faces — perhaps as a carryover from childhood or because of complexion problems during adolescence. Women patients confess that too often they go to bed at night without removing makeup, and men patients tell us that any skin care outside of washing their faces in the shower once a day is out of the question. These attitudes result from old habits, hang-ups, and plain old laziness and procrastination.

How long have you ignored simple steps or even more significant ones which could lead you toward being your best? There is no shortage of educational information. Every magazine you pick up has an article related to self-improvement. For example, information about skin care and preventing premature aging of the skin is everywhere, yet many people do not take advantage of positive and preventive information and treatment options which are available. Some of us ignore or reject these options in spite of their potential benefits. Perhaps this passive resistance is due to a lack of motivation, or ingrained attitudes about self-improvement. When it comes to issues such as aging or the dangers of sun exposure, maybe deep down you think, "It will never happen to me." Maybe you don't believe things you can't see.

We all have certain preconceived notions and stigmas which stow away in our minds. It is impossible to grow up without them. The problem comes when these ingrained attitudes and ideas stand between us and doing what it takes to be the best we can be. These same mindsets can also cause you to waste valuable time. They can actually demotivate and deactivate you.

This is why it is a good idea every once in awhile to conduct an objective evaluation of your decision-making processes. Do you make good decisions which are well thought out and based on facts, or do you sometimes make rash decisions because your mind was made up in advance?

The best approach to making decisions about what you will and will not do, can and cannot do, etc., is to remind yourself of an old expression: "The mind is like a parachute. It works better when it is open."

Slow down and try to expand your vision to all the possibilities that exist. Whether you're dealing with skin care or any other method to enhance your appearance and give you a new mindset, there are two major factors: objectivity and an open mind. Do not let a lack of education or a prejudice influence your direction. Here's a real story about how a closed mind opened up to the opportunity for self-improvement.

A woman recently came to a seminar on self-improvement which we held for employees of a large corporation. Although attendance at the seminar was voluntary, she was overtly antagonistic during the question-and-answer session of the meeting, and although no one was suggesting that she either needed or wanted to improve herself, she felt a need to proclaim, "This is the face I came into this world with, and this is the face I'm going out of this world with."

At this seminar, we were using a computerized video-imaging system which enables us to show the visual effects of certain cosmetic procedures on an individual face. This video technique is very interesting for people who want to see how their skin could look with diminished acne scars, or how their face could look with a smaller nose, fewer wrinkles, etc. We had plenty of volunteers who were anxious to participate in the imaging process, but the woman who had been so vocal stood at the back of the room and acted disinterested and aloof.

However, once she began to see the projected image of others on the computer screen, she could see the potential results projected by the video-imaging system. Her interest increased, and she began to ask a few questions. Finally when everyone else left the room, she came forward and asked to see what her face would look like with diminished acne scars.

It was rewarding to see her smile because her behavior had been so defensive, and it was obvious that she did not feel very happy with herself. Actually, when she saw the potential for improving a problem that no doubt had bothered her for a long time, her whole personality changed. Within a month's time she came to see us and seems to be very happy with her improved complexion.

In the process of improving her complexion, she decided to have her nose reshaped and some excess fat suctioned out from under her chin. She lost about thirty pounds, has a new hair style, and shows a decidedly renewed interest in life.

You Always Have a Choice

As physicians, our role is not to formulate opinions or direct decisions. We are here to present objective information and to perform appropriate medical procedures. However, we are always interested in how patients feel, not only healthwise but emotionally. The most gratifying part of our work is to see the happiness people experience when they choose to improve their appearances, to see the way self-improvement makes people feel about themselves, and to observe the many ways in which people improve their lives once they feel good about themselves.

Responsible self-improvement is not vain or selfish, nor a luxury reserved for the female sex. It does not reflect a lack of masculinity or an excess of feminine vanity. Self-improvement is for ordinary people with ordinary problems and ordinary goals. It may not be

viewed as absolutely necessary to life, but in many cases it is absolutely essential to healthy self-esteem.

So, whether you think you want to improve the quality of your skin, change something about your face or body, or improve a problem you were born with or one that has only recently surfaced, go ahead and explore the options freely. Resolve to make decisions based on objective information and patient, realistic expectations, but be sure to leave the negative ideas behind you. There's no room for those any more.

Skin Sense

In order to increase our knowledge of ourselves and to understand how to keep the single most visible organ of the body looking good and staying healthy, let's take a close look at skin — what it consists of, how it works, and how it is affected by aging and other influential factors.

The skin is the largest organ of the body. If the skin of an adult male who weighs about 150 pounds was spread out on a flat surface, it would cover about twenty square feet. Skin is responsible for waterproofing the body so that precious fluids which bathe the tissues will not be lost. It also protects the body from bacteria and chemicals that can enter the body and cause harm.

Three Layers of Skin

It is a good idea to learn the basics of skin so that you can understand how skin changes and learn to recognize many of the skin-related terms used in cosmetic applications and medical procedures. The structure of skin has two layers of tissue: epidermis and dermis, with subcutaneous tissue — which is mostly fat — for insulation. The epidermis is the outer layer which covers the entire body and is only about as thick as a single sheet of paper. The epidermis consists of four layers of cells from the outermost to the innermost: horny, granular, spinous, and basal layers.

The horny layer consists of multiple rows of dying cells which are filled with a tough, waterproof protein called keratin. The granular layer consists of one or two rows of dying cells that contain a substance called keratohyaline. The spinous layer is composed of about five to ten rows of living cells that touch one another. Finally, the basal layer, which is also made up of living cells, consists mainly of a single row of basal cells and melanocytes. These cells produce a brownish pigment called melanin. The basal cells are continually dividing. As they divide, some of the cells remain in the basal layers and some move toward the outer surface of the skin, eventually forming the upper layers of the epidermis. These upwardly mobile cells are called keratinocytes, and they produce keratin, the substance responsible for making the skin turn tough. Keratin also prevents skin from losing certain fluids and vital substances. As the keratinocytes continue the upward movement, they become filled with increasing amounts of keratin. By the time they actually reach the outer surface of the skin they are dead cells — dry flakes of skin that build up on the surface and eventually are sloughed away.

The next layer of skin is the middle layer, or the dermis, which, depending on the individual, is between 15 and 40 times as thick as the epidermis. The dermis consists mainly of blood vessels, nerve endings, connective tissue, and collagen, which is a protein that serves as the support structure for the skin. The blood vessels in the dermis nourish both the dermis itself and the epidermis. The surface of the dermis contains tiny elevations called papillae, which help connect the dermis to the epidermis. It is these papillae that contain the sensitive nerve endings that are especially numerous on the palms and fingertips. If you have ever wondered why it hurts so much to have a needle prick on your fingertip, it is because of the high degree of nerve endings contained in that tiny area.

Moving under the skin's surface, you come to the layer known as the subcutaneous tissue, which is the thickest layer. Like the dermis, its thickness varies among individuals. The subcutaneous tissue consists mainly of connective tissues, blood vessels, and cells that store fat. This layer helps protect the body from injuries such as those caused by impacts or blows, and it also helps the body retain heat. When a person overeats, it is this level of skin that increases as the body begins to store fat. It is also this layer that stores the fat that will be used when the body needs energy not available from other sources.

In addition to these three layers, the skin also includes hair, nails, and certain glands such as the sebaceous and sweat glands, which are formed from the basal cells of the epidermis or outer layer of the skin. The sebaceous glands secrete an oil referred to as sebum, which lubricates the hair and the skin's surface. The sweat glands, which produce perspiration for cooling the body, are present throughout the surface of the skin, but they are most prevalent on the forehead, palms of the hands, and soles of the feet.

What Is Collagen?

We hear a lot about collagen (the name is derived from the Greek word for glue) because recent medical advances in nonsurgical cosmetic procedures focus on the body's loss of collagen and how it can be replaced.

As already mentioned, just below the epidermis lies the dermis. Although the dermis contains blood vessels, nerve endings, and hair follicles, it is primarily made up of a protein called collagen. Because collagen is the primary component of the dermis, it acts as the support structure for the skin.

Collagen is the single most abundant protein found in humans as well as in other animals. It is the principal component of bone, cartilage, and connective tissue and gives the face

as well as the body much of its shape and substance. Fibers of collagen are woven together throughout the entire body like threads of fabric and form a framework into which new cells and blood vessels can grow.

The way your skin looks is directly related to the way in which your skin is supported. In young skin, the collagen framework is intact, and the skin remains moisturized and elastic. It is resilient to the many facial expressions we adopt and to every day wear and tear, but over time the support structure weakens and the skin loses its elasticity. Skin begins to lose its tone when collagen begins to wear down. Every time you smile, squint, laugh, or frown, you put stress on the collagen in your skin. The effect of this normal stress is cumulative and is basically what causes facial lines to begin to appear.

Injury and disease are other factors that can weaken the collagen fibers. Loss of collagen is related to the formation of wrinkles, facial lines, and creases, but today, medical advancements are providing methods for replacing collagen in order to improve these conditions. (A detailed discussion of collagen replacement appears in the sections "Soft-Tissue Augmentation" and "Collagen Replacement.")

The Color of Skin

Skin color varies among races of people and among individuals, but it is determined primarily by the amount of the brown pigment called melanin which is produced in the skin. Although people of all races have basically the same amount of melanocytes (pigment skin cells) in the epidermis which are responsible for melanin production, the melanocytes of dark-skinned people produce more melanin than those of light-skinned people. Although this process is primarily conditioned by heredity, exposure to sunlight speeds up melanin production, causing light skin to darken or tan. Melanin is also responsible for freckles, which are simply a buildup of melanin in a specific spot on the skin's surface. Obviously, sun exposure increases the production of freckles. With age, we tend to produce melanin at varying and uneven rates. This is what causes age spots or "liver" spots.

How Skin Ages

Under normal conditions, the skin actually follows a very patient approach to aging. The changes we see over the years result from a series of processes that occur very gradually over an extended period of time.

Skin begins to age at birth, which is the only time that skin is virtually perfect. Wrinkles begin to form as our facial movements repeatedly move the skin and stretch and fold it in certain patterns. It is hard to imagine, but when a baby first smiles, the stress to the skin's collagen and elastic fibers begins.

The Pull of Gravity

The next big stress factor on skin comes when we begin to pull our bodies to an upward position and crawl and then begin to walk. Gravity begins to take its toll on children as young as five or six who show signs of a downward turn at the angles of the mouth. As the pull of gravity continues, the lines become folds and get deeper and deeper.

The pull of gravity also causes the upper and lower eyelids to fall, and in some cases over time, this condition can actually impair vision. Other effects of gravity on the face include the formation of jowls. For example, there is a small fat pad in the upper cheek that makes a downward migration and eventually forms a jowl where smooth skin used to be. Gravity causes the ears and the nose to get longer. The tip of the nose begins to point toward the ground rather than straight outward. Also, frequent weight gain and loss accentuates the effects of gravity by loosening the skin and allowing it to sag even more than it otherwise would.

If you ever want to see just how much gravity has affected your facial skin, get a hand mirror and lie down on the bed with your head off the bed upside down. Look at your face in the mirror, but be prepared for a shock. Even people who are chronologically young can see how gravity has caused skin to appear loose and sagging. Now, lie on the bed flat on your back and look up at your face in the mirror. There's a big difference in appearance when when the pull of gravity is lessened.

A well-toned man in his sixties who is a bodybuilder once remarked, "I have the toned body and the agile mind of a thirty year old, but I have the wrinkled face of a sixty year old." Of course, what he's referring to is the fact that he has kept his body in terrific shape, his mind is alert and youthful, but he wants to know what happened to his face.

The truth is, there are many factors which have contributed to his aging face, including gravity and genetic factors, but it is clear that the kind of physical fitness program that tones his body and strengthens his muscles does not work in the same way on his face as it does on the rest of the body. It is not possible to decide to get your face in shape without benefit of cosmetic surgery because the damage to the structure of the face caused by sun exposure, improper diet, smoking or excessive alcohol, pollutants, and other toxic substances are irreversible.

More Free Radicals

As you recall from our previous discussion on free radicals in the chapter "Secrets of Eating Smart," these devilish free radicals are unstable molecules in our bodies which literally attack other unsuspecting molecules, setting up reactions that are damaging to other healthy cells in the body. Free radicals are created when oxygen molecules inside our bodies break down under conditions of metabolism, radiation, exercise, ozone exposure, carcinogens, and other environmental toxins.

Research indicates that the damage caused by years of free radical activity is linked to aging — and the formation of wrinkles in the skin — as well as cancer, heart disease, arthritis, emphysema,

Parkinson's disease, and over fifty other diseases. The human body's built-in repair systems cannot work fast enough to handle the continued onslaught of free radical activity. The cumulative damage to the body over time diminishes the cell's ability to make repairs. This situation is believed to be the cause of physical degeneration associated with aging.

The best available approach to this problem is prevention. Avoiding sun exposure and smoking, getting balanced amounts of nutrients from a healthy diet, and avoiding pollutants and other toxic substances can all have positive preventive impact.

Skin Sins

But now, let's take a closer look at how free radicals are linked to wrinkles. Sun damage (including UVA and UVB rays) and thermal damage are associated with free radical activity. If you are a bodybuilder, an outdoor-exercise enthusiast, a jogger, a gardener, an outdoor swimmer, or anyone who spends time in the sun getting tan or just being outdoors, chances are your skin will be prematurely aged and damaged by the sun. That means wrinkles, wrinkles, and more wrinkles — not to mention the strong possibility of skin cancer.

Skin is the first point of entry for free radicals as the harmful effects of ultraviolet light from the sun penetrate the skin. The body has a natural built-in defense system of antioxidants which to some extent can neutralize the free radicals. However, with age the natural defense system becomes less effective.

Another big skin sin is smoking. Have you ever noticed how much more wrinkled a smoker's face is than a non-smoker's face — especially if the person has been smoking for many years? Smoking causes restricted blood flow which results in nutrient deficiencies, oxygen starvation, and reduction of the body's normal processes of waste elimination. What this means to the health of your skin is that smoking impedes the body's ability to nourish the skin, short-circuits its oxygen supply, and slows down the body's ability to get rid of waste in the system.

There are certain antioxidants which protect the skin, working much like they do inside the body to combat the damaging effects of free radical activity. Typically, after the ages 35–40, the pigment cells in skin (melanocytes) begin to decrease. These cells perform the important task of fighting off free radicals responsible for inducing malignancies and combating those which destroy connective tissue beneath the skin, making way for wrinkles to form.The pigment cells provide a natural source of antioxidants to aid in this battle, but as the number of pigment cells decreases with age the amount of antioxidants decreases proportionately.

Research shows that it may be possible to provide additional antioxidants from vitamins and other substances in order to augment the diminishing supply produced by

pigment cells in older people. The major antioxidants are vitamins A, C, and E; Pycnogenol; CoQ-10; the trace mineral selenium; and the amino acid cysteine. Vitamin C is the blood supply's major antioxidant because it helps to protect blood fats from free radical attack. Vitamin E is the cell membranes' major antioxidant, and vitamin A is the major antioxidant in mucous membranes.

For detailed information on how nutrients affect the processes of the body and help protect the body against disease and aging, *The New Super Nutrition: Your Guide to Super Health and Vitality* is recommended reading. This informative book is written by Richard A. Passwater, Ph.D., and published by Pocket Books, a division of Simon and Schuster, 1230 Avenue of the Americas, New York, NY 10020.

The Environmental Factor

Many of the negative influences on skin come from areas where we have some degree of control. Exposure to air conditioning, heating systems, sunlight, heat, wind, and cold weather; changing levels of humidity; elevation; geography; airplane travel; and certain chemicals such as chlorine contribute to every skin change that occurs throughout life. Of course we cannot control the environment, but we can protect ourselves from its destructive forces with moisturizers, gentle cleansers, and sunscreens.

If you compare skin from parts of your body that are always protected from the environment, such as the underside of the breast or the lower portion of the buttocks, with skin that is constantly exposed to the elements, such as on your face or the top of your hands, you can probably see a marked difference.

Sun Damage

There has been a lot of attention paid lately to the damaging effects of the sun — both as the leading cause of skin cancer and as a major contributor to premature aging. Yet, millions of people of all ages seek out that beautiful ball of fire in the sky to bask in its warmth and soak up its radiation. In addition to the cumulative damage that may not show up until years later, the sun is breaking down collagen fibers, loosening elastic tissues, and producing wrinkle after wrinkle. The thought that a suntan is attractive is totally ironic when, in fact, a tan could be a death mask. Read on.

We encourage all young people who like to sunbathe and tan to stop and observe the skin of any person over age fifty who has spent much time in the sun. It is very valuable to create an awareness of the difference between older skin that is sun damaged and older skin that is not. The sun makes skin appear tough and weathered. This condition is sometimes referred to as sailor's skin. In an older person who has been exposed to the sun over a period of years, the appearance of the skin is rugged, tough, and deeply wrinkled with lines and creases.

In an older person whose skin is not sun damaged, the quality of the skin is softer, smoother, and much more elastic. Aging is reflected in everyone's skin, but anyone who avoids sun exposure and uses sunscreens will definitely have better-looking skin that ages much more gracefully.

Although you may think a tan makes you look good now, its lasting effects are incredibly destructive to the quality of your skin. With all the greatly improved sunless tanning products that have been developed and are readily available today, it is possible to get a tan without ruining your skin.

But not all damaging sun exposure comes from sunbathing. Sun plays a big part in all outdoor activities, and we all get sun exposure just walking in and out of our homes and offices everyday. That is why we must protect our skin with sunscreen. But it is the constant and cumulative sun exposure intensified by the decreasing protection of the earth's ozone layer that causes increasing numbers of skin-cancer cases.

Tanning Booths

Tanning booths and tanning beds are touted by their manufacturers and those who sell time in them as "safer than the sun." In reality, they are as harmful as the sun, if not worse. Their cumulative effects have caused destruction, and their use has aged the skin of everyone who has ever used one. Many people say that they go to a tanning bed before going on a beach vacation in order to get a base tan and keep from burning. A tanning bed tan cannot protect skin from burning, and there is never any safe reason to expose your skin to a tanning bed.

Here's the situation. The sun emits three bands of ultraviolet rays: band A, band B, and band C rays. UVC rays are cosmic rays that are basically kept out of the earth's atmosphere. UVB rays represent the sun's burning spectrum. UVA is the so-called tanning spectrum and is the light that is emitted by the tanning bed. The tanning bed emits 100 percent UVA — a ray that penetrates skin much deeper than UVB. As a matter of fact, UVA can penetrate harm past the skin's layers deep into the muscle. UVA also ages the skin much faster than UVB and is thought to contribute more to the development of malignant melanoma than UVB. UVA is the exact wave length which causes cataracts, and although goggles are often available, they are not always used because tanners do not want to get the "raccoon look."

Tanning beds are not regulated in most states. Even in states which do regulate them, it is difficult to monitor tanning salons and personnel to insure that warning signs are prominently displayed.

The light emitted by a tanning bed can react with various soaps and perfumes as well as with topical and oral medications to produce severe rashes.

Very importantly, UVA kills a skin cell called Langerhans cell, which protects us from viral infections such as herpes and AIDS.

Self-Tanning Lotions

In the last couple of years, products referred to as sunless or self-tanning lotions have been dramatically improved. Many of the products available today — if properly applied — offer a nice, safe indoor tan without the outdoor risks of sun damage to your skin. Proper application requires taking the time to apply the lotion smoothly and blending it consistently on the skin in order to avoid streaking and uneven coloration. It takes about three hours for the color effects to be noticeable, and the sunless tan normally lasts for several days. Many people like to use the sunless tan lotion year-round, but product literature recommends mild exfoliation between applications for smoother, more consistent results.

There are many different products on the market, and the one you like best will depend on your personal preference. It is a good idea to choose one that does not use artificial dyes and one that offers a choice of lotions for fair, medium, or dark skin. Fair-skinned people tell us that lotions formulated specifically for their skin type offer more natural-looking results. While many different products are on the market, a favorite among our staff and patients is the Estée Lauder Self-Action Tanning Creme, which is available in light, medium, and dark shades.

Proper application is crucial to getting an overall, even color on your skin. The best way to apply the lotion is after a warm bath or shower when you have exfoliated the skin with a loofa, buff-puff, or terry wash cloth. Apply a moisturizer while the skin is still wet and pat dry. Wait a few minutes until the skin has cooled from the warm bath or shower and then apply the tanning lotion. Do remember that most of the sunless tan lotions do not contain sunscreen and would thus offer no protection from sun exposure.

Skin Cancer

A variety of pigmentary changes which occur on the skin are caused by sun exposure. These changes produce irregularities on the skin such as lentigines (also known as liver spots) which are flat collections of pigment frequently found on the face and backs of hands. These often respond to treatment with Retin-A®, glycolic acid, or other medicated creams. Seborrheic keratoses are raised brown- to black-colored crusty lesions that are found mostly on the chest. They are usually harmless and can easily be removed by your doctor. Actinic keratoses are small rough patches that feel like sandpaper. Some medical experts are of the opinion that if not treated early, these actinic keratoses can lead to more serious skin conditions.

Not all skin problems are as forgiving as these pigment changes. There has been an increase in all types of skin cancers due to the popularity of suntanning and outdoor recreation. In 1992, over 650,000 people in the United States alone will develop skin cancer, and sun is the major cause. What happens is that prolonged sun exposure leads to instantaneous mutation of pigment cells in the skin. Once these cells are altered, they can become malignant.

There are three types of skin cancer: basal cell carcinoma, squamous cell carcinoma, and malignant melanoma. Basal cell carcinoma is the most common type of skin cancer and the most common cancer in general. Caused by sun exposure, basal cell carcinoma is most common on the face and hands, since these areas are most often exposed to the sun. It usually appears as a sore which does not heal and is slightly elevated from the surface of the skin. It is often characterized by a pearly gray border at the edges of the elevation with blood vessels that appear around and on top of the area. This type of cancer always starts small in size but can become quite large if left untreated. However, it rarely spreads to other parts of the body. Although a basal cell carcinoma does not invade the blood stream and move to other parts of the body in that way, it can grow extensively on the local surface of the skin, moving from an area on the face to the eye or nose with destructive and disfiguring results.

As is the case with all cancers, early detection is the best avenue toward successful treatment. There are a number of different methods currently being used to treat basal cell carcinoma. The most reliable treatment dermatologists and plastic surgeons use is to surgically extract the tumor and send it to a pathologist for a thorough examination. The pathologist has the very important role of determining that all the cancer has been removed. Other methods include freezing the cancer or scraping it out. Although these methods are used, they do not offer as precise an evaluation of cancers as the method that surgically removes and studies them.

Another surgical method is called Mohs' surgery, in which surgeons excise the tumor and examine it under a microscope as they perform the surgery. This method has specific applications for certain areas of the face, such as the corner of the eye and the corner of the nose, as well as in treatment of recurrent problems of basal cell carcinoma. Mohs' surgery is not recommended as a first line of defense because it tends to be more destructive to the remaining areas of skin. Some of the advocates of this method point out that basal cell carcinoma is itself very destructive, but it usually takes many years for the basal cell carcinoma to create the degree of damage that the Mohs' surgical method may produce in a matter of minutes. Regardless of treatment method, basal cell carcinoma cure rates approach 95 to 98 percent.

The second kind of skin cancer, squamous cell carcinoma, is less common than basal cell carcinoma. Squamous cell carcinomas appear as raised, pink opaque growths. This type of skin cancer can spread through the body especially if it is located on the lip. Squamous cell carcinomas also occur in what doctors refer to as clinically damaged skin, such as in a diabetic's leg ulcer, or from sun-damaged spots on the lips, and in the mouths of smokers or smokeless-tobacco users. It is potentially much more serious than basal cell carcinoma and is more difficult to treat.

Squamous cell carcinoma can be a problem which may vary by degrees, depending on the source of the cancer. When a squamous cell carcinoma develops from an actinic keratosis or from an overgrowth of the skin, it generally does not tend to metastasize (spread to another part of the body) and is easily treated by freezing the skin with liquid nitrogen, or treating the area with fluorouracil cream, or Retin-A.

If the squamous cell carcinoma develops from a leg ulcer or is on the vermilion border of the lip or in the mouth, a serious problem can result. The cancer must be dealt with immediately and aggressively and treated surgically in order to prevent spreading. The cure rate in squamous cell carcinoma is good in all areas except the lip which is more difficult to treat.

In most cases, squamous cell carcinoma is not caused by sun exposure so much as by trauma to the lip, such as a repeated habit of lip biting, smoking cigarettes, or using smokeless tobacco products such as snuff and chewing tobacco. The incidence of squamous cell carcinoma of the lip is on the rise among teenagers, which reflects their growing use of smokeless tobacco products. Anyone of any age should take heed that this kind of cancer can be very aggressive and that treatment can be a devastating surgery. Smokeless tobacco products must be avoided!

The third type of skin cancer is referred to as malignant melanoma. From the previous discussion, you learned that if detected and treated early, basal cell carcinoma can be successfully treated and is rarely fatal. A malignant melanoma is another story all together. Malignant melanoma has one of the fastest-growing mortality rates in the country, striking over 30,000 people in 1991, up almost 15,000 from just a decade ago. Melanoma is increasing faster than any other cancer in the United States. Today it strikes people in their twenties and thirties, whereas it used to be rare to see it in anyone under forty. In fact, this is the most common cause of cancer death in women between the ages of 20 and 25.

The Dwindling Ozone Layer

The increase in skin cancer, especially melanomas, is attributed to the disappearing protection of the earth's ozone layer. Recently the Environmental Protection Agency (EPA) announced that the earth's protective ozone layer is dwindling down twice as rapidly as previously expected. As this process continues due to the chlorofluoro-carbons and other chemicals that are destroying our environment, the incidence of skin cancer as well as other serious problems continues to rise.

The diminishing ozone layer lets in more of the sun's ultraviolet rays and is said to be the chief cause of the extreme increase in melanomas and other skin cancers. We go outside more for recreation and exercise, and exposure to sunlight is even more dangerous than it ever was because there is less natural protection.

Here's what to look for. Basal cell carcinoma develops from the cells that produce the actual layers of the skin, whereas melanoma develops from the pigment cells of the skin. A melanoma can develop from a mole that changes, from skin where no mole is present, from a dark round spot or a larger multicolored patch, and even from the pigment cells of the eye.

The only treatment for melanoma is to surgically remove it and then to send the excised specimen to a pathologist for evaluation. Early detection is essential to successful treatment. It is very important to learn what to look for in this type of skin cancer because it has the highest fatality rate of all skin cancers. The first place to watch is moles. Everyone has moles on the skin. It is important to make a mental map of the location, size, shape, and appearance of each mole on the body and to conduct a regular inspection for any changes which may have occurred.

Moles are a little collection of cells that have migrated along the skin as it is being formed before you were born.

Moles come from the same tissue that forms the brain and the spinal cord. At birth, there are rarely any moles present on the body. They begin to appear during the first year of life and continue to appear until age fifty or sixty, and then they actually begin to disappear.

Most moles are harmless, but certain moles should be examined and removed. The ones to watch closely and to show your doctor are those that change in any way — in size, shape, color — and any mole that itches, bleeds, or hurts. Also watch moles that are subject to any trauma, such as those constantly being rubbed by a bra strap or the elastic of any undergarment, or those that get constant pounding or pressure on your foot or buttocks. One of the things we do know about cancer is that trauma is associated with its development (for example, smoking traumatizes the lungs). Other suspicious moles that probably warrant removal include those which have more than one color and those which do not have a distinct border.

In cases of possible skin cancer: early detection, total removal of the cancer, and evaluation of the excised tissues by a qualified pathologists are keys to treating skin cancers successfully. An important part of the responsibility for early detection is up to each person. Charting and checking your own skin to determine changes in moles and warts, as well as being aware of unusual skin irritations and sores that resist healing and seeing your doctor immediately when you discover irregularities are essential.

The most important step to take is to consult your doctor right away if you have any questions about a mysterious mole or suspicious skin irregularity. If you do not have a doctor, The American Academy of Dermatology has skin cancer screening clinics in most cities and towns where you can be evaluated in order to determine if further attention or treatment is necessary. This screening service is provided free of charge and is open to the public.

Choosing a Dermatologist

Dermatology is the science that is concerned with the diagnosis and management of skin diseases and disorders, as well as the prevention of skin problems and the overall health of the skin, hair, and nails. Most people will, at one time or another, require the services of a dermatologist, and choosing a qualified doctor whose education, qualifications, and experience are best suited to your needs is very important.

It takes many years of specialized training to become a dermatologist. First there's undergraduate college and medical school, followed by an approved one-year internship and three-year residency program. Upon completion of this extensive curriculum, the doctor can obtain certification by the American Board of Dermatology only after passing rigorous written and oral examinations administered by extensively trained and experienced dermatologists.

The specialty of modern dermatology has many sub-specialties within its circle. There are dermatologists who specialize in cosmetic dermatology, dermatological surgery, pathology (study of skin diseases), pediatric dermatology, and Moh's surgery.

The results of dermatology treatment and the success of dermatologic surgery depend on the knowledge, skill, and experience of the dermatologist you choose. When you visit a dermatologist, talk candidly about any problem you may have, and feel free to ask questions. The best patient is one who is communicative and well informed.

If you have questions about a dermatologist's board certification or if you need assistance locating a qualified dermatologist who specializes in a certain sub-specialty, you can consult *The American Board of Medical Specialists (ABMS) Compendium of Certified Medical Specialists* or *The Directory of Medical Specialists* available at most libraries. The two professional organizations in dermatology are the American Academy of Dermatology, whose members include a broad spectrum of sub-specialties within dermatology, and the American Society for Dermatologic Surgery, whose members tend to specialize in cosmetic dermatology and dermatologic surgery. For more information or a referral service, please contact:

The American Academy of Dermatology
930 North Meacham Road
Schaumburg, IL 60196-1074

American Society for Dermatologic
    Surgery
930 North Meacham Road
Schaumburg, IL 60196-1074
(800) 441-2737 (Monday-Friday, 8:30-
    5:00 Central Standard Time)

Internal Skin Changes

Recently, studies have shown that changes occur in the skin which are independent of changes caused by the sun or other environmental factors and secondary to the effects of gravity and muscle action. These changes occur subtly and were not even discovered until recently when more sophisticated methods were developed to observe them.

Collagen and elastic fibers actually reside in a substance in the lower part of the skin known as ground substance. Ground substance consists of three very complicated molecules called acid muco-polysaccharides. They are chondroitin sulfate, hyaluronic acid, and dermatan sulfate.

Ground substance acts as a medium for the various fibers to rest in and actually serves as a glue to hold them together. It plays an important role in the condition of the skin, and scientists from pharmaceutical and cosmetic companies around the world are currently involved in extensive research to learn more about this valuable substance.

Hereditary Aging

Like longevity itself, the aging process is determined by genetics, and people age at varying rates. Although visible signs are not apparent, the actual aging process officially begins about the time the puberty stage is fully completed. The first visual differences associated with aging in the face have to do with skin's thickness and its elastic quality.

As you age, the skin area actually expands. As the skin expands, something else occurs. The skin gets thinner and begins to lose its elasticity, the quality that allows the skin to stretch out and stretch back — much like a piece of elastic or a rubber band. In addition, the ligaments that hold the muscles and skin to the facial skeleton also begin to expand. It is this process that gives the skin its sagging appearance.

Since there is little anyone can do about the ancestors who preceded them, the best advice in increasing longevity is to learn everything possible about the varying conditions that increase the rate at which aging occurs and to adjust lifestyle and habits accordingly.

Intrinsic Aging

When applied to the face, the term *intrinsic aging* simply refers to the aging that occurs by degrees. The human body is pre-programmed to get older and eventually die, and we have yet to unlock the secret that is responsible for this process. The skin, however, has the potential to outlast any other organ system of the body. Studies have been performed grafting skin from a single rat donor to successive generations of rats showing that skin could actually live for ten years, which is five times greater than the life expectancy of the animal.

Although there have only been a few human studies, there is evidence which indicates human skin can significantly outlast human life expectancy. Actually, as we age and as the biological clock slows down, the skin — if properly protected — continues to perform and keep its appearance very well. As a matter of fact, the actual aging process of skin does not play a significant role in the face until the seventh decade of life. Although some people show changes in the cells of skin as early as the third or fourth decades of life, these changes are not obvious to see. The aging changes we see are due to a loss of substance. Fat is also lost underneath the skin's surface, as well as the bony structure upon which the skin rests. Think of the oldest-looking person you have ever seen — someone over ninety or one hundred years old. The aging look you see results from skin which is literally hanging over a very thin, transparent skull.

There is treatment for intrinsic aging problems. If tissue is lost, it must be replaced. Therefore, the treatment is either fat transplantation to build up the lost tissue or silicone implantation to augment bone loss.

Sleep Lines

Did you know that the way you sleep influences the lines and creases that accumulate on your face? It's true. The sleep lines in our faces perhaps reveal more about true chronological age than any other factor. In teenagers, for instance, these lines appear during sleep and disappear shortly after arising. In thirty-year-olds, sleep lines may disappear before afternoon. In forty- to fifty-year-olds, the sleep lines may not disappear at all. Sleep lines occur for the same reasons creases occur in napkins. We push our faces into the pillow every night in relatively the same positions, creating a fold or wrinkle that remains as an indentation. Men tend to wear these lines on their foreheads, women on their cheeks. There is no set pattern which determines how these lines are formed other than the way we sleep and the stress we place on our facial structures. Changing sleep patterns is very difficult because they are habitual and unconscious, so don't stay up all night worrying about it.

Skin Vitamins

A simple, to-the-point discussion of skin vitamins is very healthy. Everyone knows that vitamins are a good thing, but do you know how they work and how they help the skin stay healthy? For example, did you know that in order to be classified as a vitamin, a substance must be found necessary in the diet in order to prevent a specific disease? This means we have to eat our vitamins in order to be healthy and keep eating them in order to prevent disease.

Vitamins are a major group of nutrients that the body needs for growth and health. They function as catalysts within the body itself. What happens is that vitamins help accelerate certain chemical reactions which the body requires in order to stay healthy. Vitamins regulate these chemical reactions and in turn help the body convert food into energy and living tissue. This is an important process for healthy skin because, as we explained, skin is constantly creating new living cells and sloughing off old, dead ones. Without essential vitamins, these important reactions would happen in the body very slowly or not at all.

There are two basic kinds of vitamins: water soluble and fat soluble. The water-soluble vitamins — including the B complex vitamins and vitamin C — dissolve in water. The fat-soluble vitamins — vitamins A, D, E, and K — dissolve in fat. The best way to obtain vitamins is to eat a balanced diet, including a variety of foods from each food group.

Many people supplement their diets with daily vitamin supplements, but it is always a good idea to consult your doctor before taking vitamin supplements to be sure you are following a program that is right for your body and your special needs. Each vitamin has specific uses in the body, one vitamin cannot replace or act for another, and the lack of one vitamin can interfere with the function of another. A continued lack of one vitamin causes a vitamin deficiency, which can lead to vitamin-deficiency diseases. Plus, randomly taking vitamin supplements may tilt the balance of vitamins in the wrong direction. If you get too much of a fat-soluble vitamin, you can create a toxic effect within the body. On the other hand, unnecessary water-soluble vitamins are eliminated through the body's natural waste process.

We know that certain vitamins and minerals play an important role in skin health. For example, vitamin C is necessary for collagen to remain strong and intact so that it can support the skin, prevent the skin from sagging, and keep blood vessels from showing through the skin's surface. Vitamin C is also helpful in tissue metabolism and wound healing.

Vitamin E helps oxygen get to the skin and allows the oxygen to be utilized properly throughout the entire body. Vitamin E is thought to promote healing and is often given after surgery as a natural edge in the healing process. However, vitamin E can cause bleeding and should not be taken prior to surgery. Topically applied, vitamin E is thought to help smooth skin and promote healing of scars and burns. It is also an important player in preserving the health of cell membranes.

The B complex vitamins serve many purposes in helping the body use important nutrients and in keeping the skin healthy. For instance, vitamin B-2 helps the body's cells use oxygen and promotes tissue repair and rejuvenation. A lack of riboflavin, or vitamin B-2, causes cracks to develop in the skin at the corners of the mouth and inflamed lips, a sore tongue, and scaly skin around the ears and nose. Vitamin B-12 and folic acid are needed to produce DNA in the body's cells. DNA carries the body's entire master plan for all cell activity. Vitamin B-12 is essential for proper development of healthy red blood cells.

Vitamin A derivatives such as Retin-A and Accutane® have played a significant role in treating both skin problems and aging skin. We will have more discussion of them in the next section.

Options for Skin Treatment

The purpose of the information presented in this section is to help you sort out and understand the wide variety of treatments and products associated with skin care, skin treatments, and medical options. Let's start with a commonly asked question: What constitutes good skin care?

Routine Skin Care

A basic skin-care regimen is recommended for everyone, regardless of age, but individual skin type and condition influence both the routine and products used. Personal care is necessary to prevent skin problems and to avoid premature skin aging. Most people are concerned with keeping skin from dehydrating, but some people have the problem of too much oil. While oily skin is a problem caused by too much oil in the skin, dry skin is a problem caused by too little water. That's why water is the best moisturizer in the world and why almost every moisturizing product lists water as its primary ingredient.

The purpose of a moisturizer is to get moisture to the skin and trap it, and all those expensive ingredients that claim wondrous benefits such as hormones, collagen, elastin, placenta, etc., may be of little or no benefit. The type of moisturizer to use for special skin types, hypersensitive skin, and problematic skin should be discussed with a doctor. With most problem-free skin, general cleansing and moisturizing — and always application of sunscreen — are the essential steps necessary to keep skin healthy and maintain its quality. Basic skin care is also necessary to prevent problems and avoid premature aging. In all cases, a daily skin-care program need not be complicated and is not dependent on expensive cosmetic products.

Problems of dry skin are usually due to the skin's inability to hold water, sun damage, or excessive skin sloughing and lack of skin replacement. In order to improve dry skin, be sure to wet the skin first before applying moisturizer or medication in a cream or lotion base.

We have found that Retin-A (with special treatment to reduce the irritating side effects) and the use of glycolic acid also help dry skin. (See the section "Glycolic Acid Peel.")

Special care is needed in winter months or in summer months where climates are severely cold and hot. During extreme climate changes, skin can become overly dry and even flaky. Some doctors who practice in extreme climate areas recommend that patients get plenty of vitamins A and D in a halibut-liver or cod-liver oil capsule which provide valuable nutrients and help to lubricate the skin.

Oily skin is due to an excessive amount of oil present in the skin. Skin can be made less oily by the application of astringents or toners which generally contain alcohol, ether, acetone, or other substances that are oil soluble. Of course, astringents and toners do not stop oil production. They only temporarily remove the oil from the skin's surface. Oily skin can be improved by treatment with Retin-A or Accutane.

Sunscreens

The advent of sunscreens is one of the greatest skin developments. Everyone of all ages needs protection from the sun every day, all year long, summer or winter, rain or shine. There are two steps in learning about sunscreens. The first is simple: apply it every day (even under makeup). Reapply it after swimming or when you perspire from exercise. The second step is to use an adequate amount of sun-protection factor or SPF. The numbers which appear after SPF (such as SPF-15) do not represent a linear graph. These numbers are on a curve with a slope which significantly changes at SPF-15, which provides the optimal level of sun protection.

Although many people go out and buy sunscreens with higher sun protection factors, SPF-15 is adequate protection so long as it is reapplied after perspiring or swimming. Sunscreens with an SPF number higher than 15, do not really provide greater protection; they only contain more chemicals. Sunscreens contain PABA, which is the sunscreen itself, but because many people are sensitive or allergic to PABA, SPF products are now available which are PABA free.

In addition, most sunscreens have determined their SPF number based on their ability to protect against UVB rays and allow UVA rays to be selectively absorbed as the numbers get higher (SPF 30, 40, etc.). UVA rays are dangerous. So, by selecting a sunscreen with a number higher than 15, you may actually be exposing your skin to the worst part of the sun's rays.

Everyone, with the exception of true albinos, has some degree of natural sun protection. Sunscreen simply increases your natural sun protection ability. For example, if your unprotected skin will burn in the sun in the first 15 minutes of exposure and your neighbor's unprotected skin will burn after 30 minutes of the same sun exposure, and both of you apply a sunscreen with SPF-4, you will burn in one hour and your neighbor will burn in two hours. In other words, your natural sun protection is multiplied by the sun-protection factor of the sunscreen you apply.

The Skin Is a Working Machine

Think of the skin as a working machine that is constantly renewing itself. The cell renewal process that we explained in the previous section "Three Layers of Skin," described how a cell climbs from the bottom layer of skin to the top layer and drops off or sloughs itself away. This sloughing process of dead cells is what eventually ends up as the ring in your bathtub after you've had a bath, but the whole process of cells climbing through the layers of skin actually takes about 28 to 30 days in normal, young skin and as long as 60 or more days in people over age sixty.

A decrease in cell activity is linked to poor vascularization and blood circulation, so nutrition, exercise, and fitness play an important role in skin health. When cell activity slows down, one of the first telltale signs is dry, scaly, rough skin. It is important to keep this process running efficiently because it is this constant source of renewal that keeps skin looking fresh and feeling smooth. Avoid anything that impedes the sloughing away of dead cells because this process is essential to the rejuvenation and health of the skin.

Certain substances applied to skin actually coat the skin and slow down its natural sloughing process and cause skin to feel dry. Mixtures in products such as certain refined hydrocarbons found in mineral oils can form a film on the skin, blocking pores and interfering with normal skin respiration, and may even cause blemishes to occur.

Products containing solvent alcohol (propyl, isopropyl) have a very drying effect on the skin. Products containing artificial colors and fragrances have been known to cause allergic reactions and photosensitivity in some people, as have some animal products such as lanolin, which comes from sheep.

Soap-free cleansers which cleanse by emulsification rather than by detergent are milder than soap and gentler on skin. If you ever use a soap to cleanse the skin, be sure you choose one that is nonalkaline. Steer clear of washing your face, bathing, or showering with deodorant soaps because they are very drying. Do not use harsh brushes or rough scrub pads on skin. Facial skin is especially sensitive, but no skin likes the rough treatment. Always handle your skin with care, stroking it in gentle upward motions. Do not pull or stretch skin while cleaning or moisturizing it. If you like to use a wash cloth, those which are made of 100 percent cotton are probably less likely to cause an allergic reaction. If you like using skin-toner products, look for one that is mild and alcohol free.

Usually light-weight moisturizers will not clog pores or interfere with the natural sloughing action. Moisturizers should be applied to both face and body when wet because the water on the skin's surface helps the moisturizer to be absorbed into the skin.

Unless your skin is very sensitive, mild exfoliation is a good way to stimulate sloughing, but exfoliation should typically be performed only about once a week.

A Good Foundation

People always have questions about cosmetic foundations, which are widely used by women and sometimes by men too. For years women have used foundations to add color to their complexions and to conceal blemishes, imperfections, and irregularities. Today many men use light concealers too, which when applied with a soft sponge can lightly even out ruddiness and hide the unsightly redness of broken capillaries and other blemishes.

There is nothing wrong with using foundation, and in some cases, foundation may even protect the skin from sun as well as other elements. It is important to clean foundation and all makeup from the skin before bed and to use a foundation that feels and looks good on your skin. When purchasing a foundation, shop where you can sample a type of foundation before you have to buy a whole bottle. That way if you do not like the product, you will have one less little jar or bottle to add to your collection.

Blackheads and Whiteheads

Blackheads and whiteheads are complexion problems that can plague teenagers and adults alike. They are unsightly blemishes on the skin which no one wants to have.

Essentially, a blackhead is an open pore with a plug in it. The plug consists of hardened skin which is a protein substance. As you know, when you expose protein to air it oxidizes and turns dark. So blackheads are not dark because of dirt. They are dark from the same oxidation process that turns a slice of apple or banana dark when exposed to air.

Whiteheads are also plugged pores with oil accumulating underneath the plug. The difference is that whiteheads develop when pores are so clogged that no air can enter.

Both blackheads and whiteheads are a real nuisance and can be difficult to treat. Cleaning the surface of the skin or applying certain chemicals to the skin will not unplug the pore. However, masques can be effective against blackheads because they harden on the skin's surface and create a drying effect which stimulates a pulling action that works on the blackhead to unplug it.

There are medical treatments which your doctor can prescribe including use of Retin-A topical cream. This vitamin A derivative encourages the sloughing action which helps to unplug stubborn blackheads. A doctor or expert esthetician can perform manual extraction of blackheads which will also unclog the blocked pores.

Treating Break-Outs and Preventing Scars

During childhood the skin has tight pores, a silky feel, and a velvet touch. With the onset of puberty between the ages of 9 and 11, male hormones (which are present in both males and females) stimulate the sebaceous glands to grow larger and produce more oil. This situation can result in clogged pores producing blackheads or whiteheads, as well as small, pus-filled pimples or tender red cysts. These pimples and cysts are aggravated by a germ called Proprionobacterium acnes that is found near the hair below the skin's surface. Cysts can leave permanent scars, but pimples do not usually scar unless they are squeezed and irritated.

Boys are generally more troubled by acne than girls, but it is a problem for both sexes and a problem that can last into adulthood. Acne may be stimulated by sun exposure, stress, certain foods, and personal habits. A balanced diet, plenty of regular sleep, and exercise are helpful, but the best cure for acne is actually aging.

In recent years, food has been found not to play a significant role in the development of acne. The old thinking that chocolate and fatty foods, milk and soda contribute to acne are simply not true. However, eating large amounts of seafood with high iodine content or drinking alcoholic beverages can increase the redness associated with acne. Some acne patients do complain that certain foods trigger acne break-outs. The best advice is to stay away from anything which you feel contributes to the problem.

The basic cause of acne is a plugged oil gland, an inherited condition which is affected by changing hormone levels.

Emotions can aggravate acne too, as can certain environmental conditions such as physical exposure to "greasy" environments, (working in an auto mechanic shops or in a kitchen where a lot of food frying occurs).

In addition to cleansing the face, using benzoyl peroxide washes, which are available as over-the-counter medications, can improve the acne problem. They kill germs that live in the oil glands, help to unstop pores, and reduce oil. Choose a 5 to 10 percent benzoyl peroxide wash. Some products have a higher percentage of benzoyl peroxide, but stronger is not necessarily better. The stronger percentage may irritate the skin and in the process, close the opening to the oil glands and aggravate the situation rather than improve it. You may increase the strength of the product over time, but be sure to start with a mild solution at first and increase strength gradually.

Today there are very effective medical treatments which improve acne. These treatments require a visit to a dermatologist who is experienced in acne treatment. In most cases, prescription medications such as the antibiotic tetracycline and the vitamin A derivatives Retin-A and Accutane require careful, close medical observation and evaluation.

Retin-A

Retin-A speeds the natural cell-turnover process by loosening the super-ficial, dead-cell layer of the skin. The topical prescription medication referred to as Retin-A, (the trade name for Retinoic Acid, manufactured by Ortho Laboratories) has been on the market for about twenty years. It has been used successfully to treat acne and is also effective in improving the fine lines associated with aging skin; the brown spots, dryness, discolorations, and fine lines caused by sun damage; and the tiny red lines which are due to broken blood vessels below the skin's surface. Although first used to treat acne, patients noticed that one of Retin-A's side effects was younger-looking skin.

Retin-A has been used very effectively to treat various skin conditions. We have found Retin-A to be effective treatment in cases where pigmentation is irregular and in improving stretch marks in various areas of the body which have been caused by skin being stretched beyond its elastic capacity. Stretch marks are fractures of the skin which develop in the lower layer of the dermis and are characterized by reddish-purple, slightly depressed lines.

Treatment with Retin-A initially causes varying degrees of redness, scaly dry skin, and skin irritation, especially during the first few weeks of treat-ment. These side effects normally diminish as the skin becomes accustomed to the medication. Retin-A also causes the skin to be sensitive to sun exposure, so it is necessary to avoid excess sun exposure and carefully apply sunscreen when using the medication.

We traditionally follow a

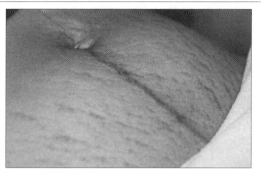
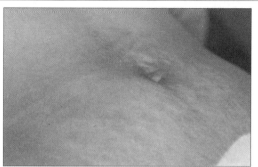

Before Retin-A treatment for stretchmarks on the abdomen

After Retin-A treatment for stretchmarks on the abdomen

treatment course starting with Retin-A Cream 0.025%, progressing to 0.05%, and finally to 0.1%, if necessary. It is impor-tant to build up exposure to Retin-A by starting with a lower-percentage solution cream and gradually increasing the percentage of Retin-A solution.

If you are interested in Retin-A, find a doctor who is both qualified and experienced in treating skin conditions and in prescribing Retin-A. We have our patients follow a certain routine which helps eliminate some of the associated irritating side effects. It is important to note that in order to get results from Retin-A, it must be used consistently and over an extended period of time. Retin-A is not a start-stop treatment. It becomes a part of your daily cleansing and moisturizing program.

Retin-A Routine

1. Wash the face with a nonirritating cleanser every morning (Cetaphil, Neutrogena liquid soap, etc.).

2. Apply sunscreen with an SPF of 15 or greater before applying makeup or foundation.

3. Wash the face with a non-irritating cleanser at bedtime.

4. Leave the face wet after cleansing.

5. Apply a small amount of Retin-A (about the size of a dime) over the entire face. Stop the application at the jawline. Avoid both upper and lower eyelid areas.

6. Moisturize. (The moisturizer Catrix®, manufactured by Donell DerMedex, is a specially formulated moisturizer developed to counteract the irritating side effects of Retin-A.) It contains a PABA-free SPF-15 sunscreen and is available through physicians only. We have found Catrix to be effective in preventing and treating the peeling and tautness some patients experience using Retin-A. For more information about Catrix, contact:

Catrix® is a registered trademark of Donell DerMedex.

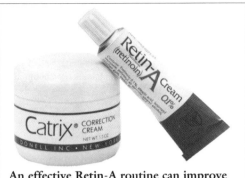

An effective Retin-A routine can improve the quality of the skin

Donell DerMedex
Suite 1422
342 Madison Avenue
New York, NY 10171
(800) 526-3461

Retin-A Myths

1. If you use Retin-A, you can never go in the sun again. **Wrong.** As long as you use sunscreen, normal sun exposure is tolerated.

2. Retin-A increases the risk of skin cancer. **Wrong.** Most skin cancer is due to sun damage, and Retin-A helps to reduce sun damage.

3. Retin-A causes birth defects. **Wrong.** The confusion here may be with another vitamin A derivative called Accutane, which is given by mouth as a treatment for severe acne. Accutane has been shown to cause birth defects — but only if you are pregnant when taking the drug. Retin-A is a topical medication (used only on the surface of the skin), and no birth defects have ever been reported in the twenty years it has been in use.

4. By drying the skin, Retin-A makes the skin age faster. **Wrong.** The drying effects of Retin-A are not necessary for it to work. Retin-A stimulates the natural cell-turnover process and increases the loosening of the dead superficial cell layer. Besides, dryness does not cause aging.

5. If you start using Retin-A and stop, your skin will look worse than it did in the beginning. **Wrong.** If you stop using Retin-A, you merely lose the benefit you have obtained thus far. You must use Retin-A consistently in order to continue obtaining results.

Dermabrasion

The skin is a multilayered structure, and there are two procedures that remove the top layer of skin so that a new, healthy surface can grow in its place: dermabrasion (see the section "Scar Wars") and chemical peel (discussed in the next section). In many cases, doctors use these two procedures interchangeably and in varying degrees to treat numerous conditions. Generally, dermabrasion is used to treat acne scars and chemical peel is used to treat wrinkles, but the final decision of whether to use dermabrasion or chemical peel depends on the individual doctor and the patient's condition.

Dermabrasion, or the "sanding" of the skin, smooths scars and reduces skin-

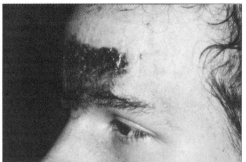

Before dermabrasion: Patient had trauma scar resulting from auto accident

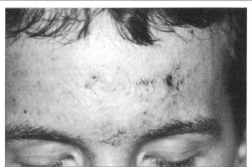

One month after dermabrasion

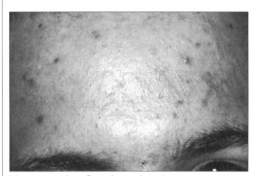

Two months after dermabrasion

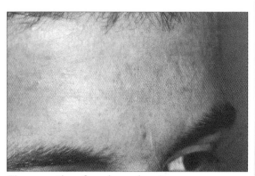

Five months after dermabrasion

surface irregularities by equalizing the margins of the scar and eliminating any elevations so that low areas in the skin's surface appear less deep. In the process of removing the top layer of skin and making way for new skin to grow in its place, it can also improve wrinkles, fine lines, and abnormal pigmentation caused by sun damage and aging. Here's how it works.

Dermabrasion involves the removal of the epidermis and some of the superficial dermis layer of the skin, while preserving enough deep layers of the skin to allow resurfacing of the dermabraded areas to occur. The sanding of the skin is performed with a mechanical abrader, a high-speed rotary wheel similar to a very fine grained sandpaper.

The procedure is performed under either local or general anesthesia. Local anesthesia numbs the area to be treated, and general anesthesia allows the patient to sleep through the entire procedure. Dermabrasion normally takes about 30 to 45 minutes and is typically performed on an out-patient basis, which means the patient goes home after the procedure to recuperate rather than staying in the hospital.

Following the procedure, the dermabraded areas are very red and sensitive, but this irritation usually subsides after a few days and can be covered with makeup. Once healing has occurred, the skin's surface is smoother, and scarred areas are less noticeable.

Chemical Peel

This procedure is also called chemabrasion, and it has a long and interesting history. It was first referred to as skin peeling, having found its way to the Unites States from Europe in the early 1900s where it was a nonmedical treatment thought to improve the quality of skin.

In the 1940s, clinics and face-peeling parlors claiming to have secret formulas for improving sun-damaged and wrinkled skin sprang up around the country, and although the medical community was aware of the activity, skin peeling was still a procedure being performed outside the supervision of medicine and without government approval. It was not until the 1950s that reputable physicians and surgeons became involved in this process. Dr. Thomas Baker, a distinguished Miami plastic surgeon, was instrumental in investigative work which resulted in securing the so-called secret "phenol" formula for skin peeling that is the basis of the chemical peel procedure widely used today. Although the formula for chemical peel is basically the same, the conditions under which the procedure is performed and the level of patient care are dramatically improved today.

A Los Angeles dermatologist, Dr. Samuel Ayres III, has been instrumental in advocating another type of chemical peel procedure using a trichloroacetic

acid peel, which is also an effective treatment in certain cases involving wrinkles and skin irregularities. Trichloroacetic acid is preferred by some doctors because in certain cases it may have fewer side effects.

Chemical peel is widely used today on the face to treat wrinkles and lines such as those which appear as horizontal lines on the forehead, lines around the eyes such as crow's feet, and creases around the mouth and above the lips. It is also used to improve abnormal pigmentation, blemishes, broken blood vessels, keratosis, and scars resulting from acne, chicken pox or minor superficial wounds.

Varying degrees of peeling are used according to the degree of the problem needing correction. A light peel is used to remove superficial wrinkles, and a deep peel is used to improve more severe skin conditions. Chemical peel on parts of the body other than the face can be very dangerous because non-facial skin, including that on the neck, does not have the physical capacity for healing and cell regrowth that the face does.

Chemical peel uses a specially formulated solution that is applied to the problem areas and actually burns away the top layers of skin. During this procedure, the patient is usually mildly sedated to ease discomfort and anxiety. There is a slight burning sensation associated with the initial application of the solution, but this diminishes quickly because the solution itself contains an anesthetic which has a numbing effect on the skin. Within 24 hours, a crust or

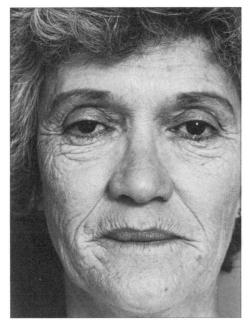
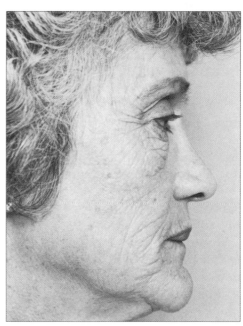

Before chemical peel

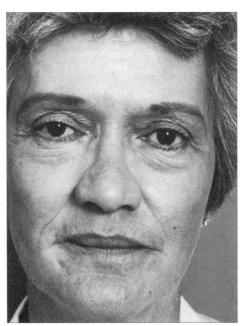
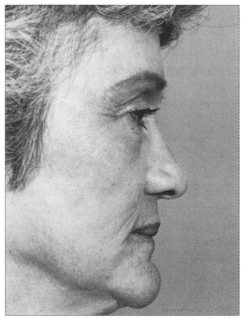

Four months after chemical peel

scab will form to protect the new skin that has been exposed at the surface. This crusty layer will eventually slough away, leaving the skin a red color similar to a bad sunburn. The healing period takes several weeks to several months, depending on the degree of the peel, but generally the post-peel period is characterized by itching, tingling, and mild discomfort which is controllable with medication.

Gradually, as healing happens over the next few days and weeks, the new skin will lighten from red to pink. Although final results may take several months to surface completely, peeling the skin results in the creation of a new layer of skin that is younger, healthier, and smoother looking than the skin that was previously in its place.

Chemical peel is also used in conjunction with or as an adjunct to facelift because the two procedures accomplish two different sets of results. A facelift is a surgical procedure (discussed in detail in the section "Facelift") which involves lifting away the skin from the deeper tissues of the face. Results of facelift include improved facial and neck contours, but a facelift does not improve or eliminate wrinkles, lines, scars, pigmentation abnormalities, or skin irregularities. In order to improve contours and correct the quality of skin, both procedures may be required.

Chemical peel and facelift can be performed at the same time only if there are small facial areas, such as around the lips or on the forehead, to be peeled. The facelift operation depends on the full forces of the blood supply for proper healing, and extensive chemical peeling could compromise that process. If more extensive peeling is involved, the peel should not be scheduled until three or four months after a facelift so that the skin has properly healed from the surgery.

Glycolic Acid Peels

Glycolic acid, also known as hydroxyacetic acid, is the simplest of a group of naturally occurring acids which are collectively known as alpha hydroxy acids, or AHAs. Many of these acids are found in natural sources such as fruit and other foods. Glycolic acid is found in sugar cane. Acids commonly known as the fruit acids include citric acid from citric fruits, malic acid from apples, lactic acid from sour milk, and tartaric acid from grapes.

Glycolic acid is used successfully in a skin-peeling procedure which improves such conditions of the skin as wrinkles, age spots, and acne. While the formulation of products and procedural techniques have been dramatically improved, the use of glycolic acids is hardly new.

In ancient Egypt, Cleopatra knew of the benefits of the alpha hydroxy or fruit acids. She used them to smooth her face and bathed in them to smooth her body. In ancient Rome, women salvaged the thick layer of acid that formed at the bottom of wine barrels while wine was aging. They applied this acid to their faces to smooth and beautify their skin. For centuries, women have used lemon juice, which is a citric acid, to lighten the skin and blend dark spots.

Glycolic acid is the simplest in structure of all the alpha hydroxy acids. It is believed that glycolic acid, because of its smaller molecular size, has the greatest penetration potential of any of the AHAs, and it is also thought to have the greatest benefit to the skin.

When glycolic acids are used as a facial peel, studies show that they help to loosen or break up the thick outer horny layer of skin where excessive buildup of dead skin cells occurs. This loosening or breaking up of the outer skin layer leads to a sloughing of dead skin cells, which in turn has proven effective for clearing and cleaning pores in acne-prone skin, smoothing fine lines in aging skin, smoothing the texture of sun-damaged skin, relieving dry skin, improving discoloration, and diminishing the unattractive appearance of broken blood vessels.

Glycolic peels are sometimes used instead of Retin-A, especially in cases where a patient's skin is continuously sensitive to Retin-A. Often a mild glycolic acid lotion is used in conjunction with the peel procedure. Patients apply daily applications of the lotion as part of the treatment process. There is no downtime or out-of-work time associated with glycolic acid peels because the results occur slowly over time, but ongoing treatments are required for good results.

Soft-Tissue Augmentation

Researchers and scientists have searched for many years for a biological material (derived from the human body or an animal or plant source; not man-made) that could be compatible with body tissues and effectively used to contour certain defects such as scars and wrinkles. A compatible biological material would ideally be able to be injected into the body without allergic reaction and could be absorbed and destroyed by the body's natural defenses should an allergic response occur.

Extensive study of the protein in our skin and connective tissue led us to understand that this protein substance, collagen, is responsible for providing the structural support for our skin, cartilage, muscles, tendons, and bones. In the case of a wound, collagen is produced by the tissue cells to help connect and bind the edges of the skin back together and produce healing. And as we get older, it is the gradual loss of our natural supply of collagen that causes wrinkles, creases, and sagging skin. Every smile, frown, or squint puts stress on and weakens the collagen supply. With this knowledge, the search was on to find a biological replacement for the body's own collagen.

In the early 1970s, a group of biochemists and physicians at Stanford University were researching alternatives to skin grafts. In the course of their work, they developed the concept of purifying animal collagen, in particular bovine (cow) collagen so thoroughly that it could be used to replace lost human collagen.

The collagen in human skin is very similar to bovine collagen, which has been used in many medical applications over the years, such as sutures and heart valves used in surgical procedures. Research and development by Collagen Corporation of Palo Alto, California, led to a family of products which use bovine collagen as an injectable implant for the repair and recontouring of aging or damaged human tissue.

The collagens manufactured by Collagen Corporation to be used for cosmetic purposes are called Zyderm® Collagen and Zyplast® Collagen. They have been used to treat approximately 700,000 people worldwide and are available for use in 28 countries.

Collagen Corporation has been involved in extensive research and development and has been amassing clinical data on their product since 1978. The substance was approved by the Food and Drug Administration (FDA) in 1981.

This type of soft-tissue augmentation is performed by a doctor who is trained and experienced in the procedure. It is typically performed by dermatologists and plastic surgeons whose practices include a specialization in cosmetic procedures.

Because a small number of people may have existing allergies and antibodies for bovine collagen (which may be the result of an acquired allergy to beef protein through dietary exposure), it is necessary to do a series of skin tests in order to determine if a patient is an appropriate candidate for injectable collagen. The procedure usually takes less than an hour and is performed in the doctor's office or surgicenter.

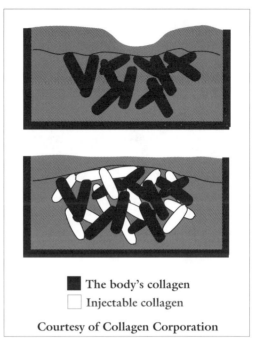

■ The body's collagen
□ Injectable collagen

Courtesy of Collagen Corporation

The bovine collagen that is used as replacement for human collagen has been scientifically purified. It is kept suspended in a saline (natural salt water) solution until it is used. It is injected through a very small hypodermic needle, and no anesthesia is required. Minor defects can be corrected in a single treatment session, but some conditions require two or more treatment sessions, depending on the size of the deformity. After treatment there is some redness and lumpiness which usually occurs in the injected areas, but this reaction normally goes away within a few days.

Once the replacement collagen has been injected into the body, the material warms to body temperature, becomes stationary, and is fixed within the tissues. Once the collagen has been in place for a few weeks, the injected areas have the

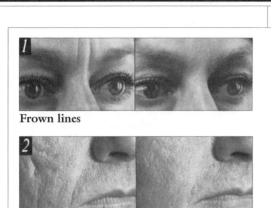

Frown lines

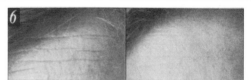

Worry lines

Acne scars

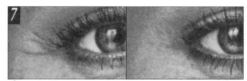

Crow's feet

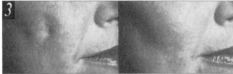

Cheek depression

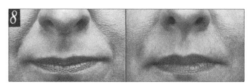

Deep smile lines

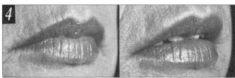

Smoker's lines

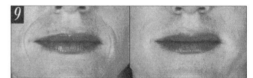

Smile lines

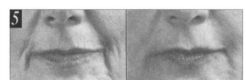

Marionette lines

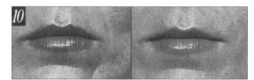

Facial scars

Courtesy of Collagen Corporation

appearance of normal skin. As a matter of fact, under a microscope, the collagen implant forms a latticework of fibers that is similar to the normal collagen framework within the skin.

For more than 700,000 people treated since 1976, injectable collagen has proven to be safe. A very small number of patients have shown an allergic reaction after one or more skin tests. Reactions such as redness, swelling, itching, and firmness at all or some of the injected areas tested have occurred, but these reactions are rare and usually only temporary.

With proper monitoring of the skin tests, many of these reactions can be avoided. Clinical data indicates that reactions to bovine collagen are specific to bovine collagen; human collagen is not affected.

Uses for Injectable Collagen

Soft-tissue augmentation with injectable collagen is widely used to fill in lines, creases, wrinkles, scars, or pox marks. It does not replace cosmetic surgery because they accomplish two different results. Cosmetic surgery such as a facelift, for instance, improves the contours of the face and tightens skin, muscles, and tissue and removes fat. A patient who has had a good result from a facelift will have smoother, firmer skin on the face and neck.

However, the facelift procedure will not correct wrinkles, lines, creases, or scars. Very often soft-tissue augmentation will be used in conjunction with facelift surgery in order to obtain the desired results of both procedures.

Collagen Replacement Therapy[SM] is used in numerous areas of the face to soften the surface of the skin and to smooth away lines and wrinkles. For example, collagen can be used to improve the tiny lines above the top lip which are referred to as perioral lines or "smoker's lines." Smokers get these lines above the top lip from drawing on a cigarette, and many nonsmokers get them from repeatedly pursing their lips. Perioral lines are also the cause of "lipstick bleed" (lipstick running into the creases above the lip), and collagen replacement can improve on this condition by smoothing out the surface and removing the creases into which the lipstick bleeds.

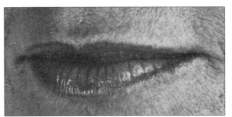

Female lips (age 40) with visible lipstick bleed lines

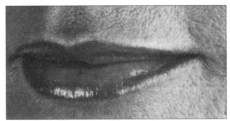

Collagen has been injected into the dermis of the skin of the lip and along the lip margin

Another use for Collagen Replacement Therapy is in oral commissures, or frown lines. These facial lines are usually caused by repeated facial expressions which cause stress and wear down the skin's natural collagen supply. Typically, they are an extension of the much deeper nasolabial folds that extend from the tip of the nose to the corners of the mouth. Mild versions of oral commissures look like small commas at the corners of the mouth. More pronounced oral commissures can extend to the chin, causing additional vertical lines that give the appearance of a "marionette's chin." Injectible collagen is also used to soften and smooth worry lines across the forehead, crow's feet at the corners of the eyes, and smile lines around the mouth.

Like the skin's natural collagen, the injected collagen begins to lose its form

Collagen Replacement Therapy[SM] is a service mark of the Collagen Corporation.

121

and will eventually wear down. In most cases where patients want to maintain good results, two to four treatments per year are required in order to maintain those results indefinitely. If you think you would like to improve facial wrinkles, lines, creases, or scars with Collagen Replacement Therapy, be sure to discuss the results you hope to accomplish with your doctor. Individual age, skin condition, amount of sun damage, and skin type will influence both the treatment and outcome of therapy.

Collagen Creams

Many creams and moisturizers containing collagen are available. Some of the advertising and literature which has appeared suggests that the topical application of collagen cream to the skin's surface can result in the absorption of collagen into the skin and that lost collagen can be supplemented. No scientific evidence has been shown to support the fact that collagen can penetrate through the skin's surface or be absorbed through the skin. Creams and moisturizers primarily slow the rate of water loss from the skin and help keep the skin's surface supple.

Scar Wars

We have mentioned the emotional effects of scars caused by acne and injury, but let's take a closer look at what causes scars and what can be done about them. One of the first questions is, What causes some injuries to scar when others do not?

As you may remember from previous discussions about the composition of skin, you are born with a uniform layer of collagen that forms a network of fibers which come together under one smooth, flexible sheath just below the surface of the skin. This layer of collagen has a lot to do with whether or not an injury or wound will form a scar and how the scar will look.

For example, a paper cut does not produce a scar. The reason is that the cut penetrates only the outer layers of skin and does not disrupt the collagen fibers which serve as the support structure for the skin itself. A sunburn damages the skin but does not produce a scar because the redness that occurs is due to the increased blood flow through the blood vessels beneath the collagen. The skin becomes red and swollen, but the collagen layers are left intact.

The reason skin scars is because there is a disturbance of the continuous fibers of collagen underneath the skin's surface. For example, when a knife or sharp object penetrates the skin and gets into the collagen layers, the collagen layer will repair itself, but the repair is never perfect. The collagen that grows back is not the same as it was before it was torn. The fibers are crooked and form a mesh-like pattern, which is the body's way of providing firmness and strength for the injured area.

As the repair process occurs, the fibers of collagen pull on the surface of the skin in an effort to close the opening. This pulling-together action causes the surface of the skin to dip down and form what looks like a crater. This functional but imperfect-looking repair job is what you see as a scar which remains after the wound or injury has healed. Sometimes when the collagen gets over zealous in its frenzy to reknit the broken areas of skin, it can produce what is known as a keloid, a scar that is unusually thick. Certain types of skin, such as olive, black, and Oriental skin, tend to scar and keloid more than other types of skin.

Also, certain diseases such as acne and chicken pox cause scars to form where trauma to the skin creates a disturbance in the collagen layer. The more severe the process of the disease, the more severe the scarring usually is. Acne produces some degree of scarring in approximately 20 percent of people who suffer from it, and it is estimated that some thirty million Americans have acne scarring as a result of the disease. Treatment of skin cancer may also result in scars, particularly in areas of the body exposed most often to the sun.

Treatment of scars depends on the size, depth, location, and the number of scars present. Dermabrasion is one of the most common methods used to improve scars. (See the "Dermabrasion" section above.) The modern procedure is attributed to Dr. Abner Kurtin, a Chicago dermatologist who tired of attempting to use manual sanding procedures to smooth out his patients' skin irregularities. Consulting with a dentist, Dr. Kurtin attached the sandpaper to a dental drill to rotate the paper, save his fingers, and improve the sanding procedure. Over the years, dermabrasion has been greatly improved, especially by the work of dermatologists

Dr. Norman Orentreich of New York City and Drs. Eugene Farber and John Yarborough of New Orleans, who have worked to perfect the procedure and have vastly improved its results.

Dermabrasion works by going past the level of the scar down to a new and fresh bundle of collagen fibers so that the skin has an improved chance of growing back smoother. In the hands of a qualified doctor who is experienced in this procedure, dermabrasion can be an effective method of improving scars, but the procedure is only as good as the doctor who is performing it, so select your doctor carefully. (See the section "Choosing Your Doctor.")

There are several schools of thought about which type of anesthesia should be used to keep the patient comfortable so that the doctor can perform dermabrasion effectively. The size of the area to be dermabraded determines the type of anesthesia used. Local anesthesia with sedation works well for smaller areas, but in some cases, larger areas may require general anesthesia. Also, by freezing the surface of the skin to be dermabraded the skin is not so contoured or pliable as it is in its normal state. Generally, the doctor performing the procedure can get better results working on "stiff" skin rather than on skin which is loose and flexible. Doctors make this comparison: Working on cooled skin is like sculpting hard ice cream as opposed to sculpting jello. The stiffened skin is less likely to be accidentally gouged and scarred.

Another great advance used in treating scars is the advent of biosynthetic dressing used in the dermabrasion procedure. Prior to the development of this type of dressing, it could take up to three weeks for the dermabraded areas to heal sufficiently so that a patient could return to work or normal social activities. With these special dressings, the healing time is greatly reduced, and although redness remains for a while longer, the crust that forms over the healing areas goes away much more quickly. Today most patients can return to work or social activities at the end of one week. Also, the use of Retin-A for a prescribed period before dermabrasion can speed up the healing process and improve results. (See the section "Retin-A.")

The timing of scar treatment with dermabrasion is also important. Dr. John Yarborough has developed a technique known as Programmed Dermabrasion which is used following multiple facial traumas caused by automobile accidents or cancer surgery. This treatment usually begins during the healing process as the collagen fibers are beginning to align themselves (usually between four to eight weeks after the trauma occurs), and results can be very good. Sometimes a doctor may advise waiting until the injury has completed healed before treatment or revision occurs, but this advice does not necessarily apply to dermabrasion.

As is the case with all procedures, treatments, and medications, there are some side effects associated with dermabrasion, and it is a very good idea for patients to understand what those side effects can be before deciding to have dermabrasion performed. The most common one is the development of milia, or small stopped-up oil glands, which occur as a result of the dermabrasion healing process.

After dermabrasion, cell regeneration occurs from the deepest level of the dermabrasion in the cells which line the pores of the skin. During this process some of the oil glands get stopped up. It is necessary, then, to go back and open up each one of the little bumps which result. This is easy to do, is painless, and produces no scars, but it is nonetheless aggravating to a person who is anxious to improve his or her skin as quickly as possible.

In rare cases acne may be reactivated after dermabrasion, but these cases do not often happen. In some other incidents, scars can be caused by dermabrasion, especially in areas where bones are close to the surface of the skin, such as the area where you cross over the jawline and cheek prominences. Pigment problems have occurred from dermabrasion, but problems involving too much pigment are treatable, and problems of too little pigment are usually temporary and very rare. Chemical peel has been used to improve scars but is generally regarded as more effective in treatment of sun-damaged skin and fine lines and wrinkles on the face. (See "Chemical Peel.")

In certain types of scars, especially scars that have the appearance of an ice-pick wound, surgical revision and skin grafting may be necessary to obtain results. When you consider that a scar is an abnormal formation in the first place, it makes sense to go to the source of the problem, the collagen framework, and consider treating the scar with injectable collagen. The general rule of thumb is when you pull on the edges of a scar and it improves, then collagen injections will most likely be able to improve the cosmetic appearance of that scar. Collagen replacement is temporary, and collagen will have to be reinjected periodically to maintain results. When collagen is used to improve scars — like those caused by acne — the results last longer than in other applications because acne scars are static; they do not move around like areas of wrinkles and lines formed in the skin, which are caused by repeated smiling, frowning, and various facial expressions. (See "Soft-Tissue Augmentation.")

In the case of acne and other types of scars, a combination of treatments may be used. For example, Retin-A can be used to prepare the skin, derma-brasion to smooth the skin, small punch grafting to correct certain ice-pick type scars, and collagen injections to fill in broader and deeper scars. Although treatments to correct scars must be appropriately timed and accomplished over a period of time, there are many excellent ways to get good results.

Working with a Professional Esthetician

Many dermatologists and plastic surgeons work in tandem with an esthetician, an experienced, licensed skin-care and cosmetics expert. After cosmetic surgery, the doctor may recommend one or several visits to this professional. Estheticians perform facial cleansings before and after surgical procedures and help patients maintain good skin-cleansing and skin-care practices. They have training and experience in specialized post-operative procedures which can promote the natural healing process and hide temporary bruising and discoloration. By skillfully applying camouflage makeup, for instance, estheticians can help patients return to work and their normal routine earlier than if they had to wait until all bruising and discoloration completely disappear.

Estheticians also work with physicians to help patients with complexion disorders to improve the condition of their skin. Keeping skin clean and keeping pores unclogged is very important to the person who suffers with acne and other complexion problems. Since acne affects teenagers most often, the esthetician can help the young person learn about and practice proper skin care and establish lifelong healthy skin-care habits. For men and women of all ages, the professional esthetician is a valuable resource for achieving and maintaining an attractive appearance and healthy skin.

Hair Today, Gone Tomorrow

This old joke may be amusing to some-one who has hair, but for the man or woman who is worried about hair loss, this is no laughing matter. Our society equates a full, healthy head of hair with youth and virility. Most of us don't even like it when our hair turns gray, but when hair starts thinning or growing in the wrong places, we get very serious about what might be done. Ironically, the problem of hair is most annoying because it seems to grow when and where we don't want it much more easily than when and where we do want it.

The most serious concerns over hair involve the growth or lack of growth on the scalp and the face, but hair growth on other parts of the body may cause serious concern for some people. The stigmas associated with hair contribute to the problem. According to tradition, a man with a beard is considered masculine, but excess facial hair on a woman is undesirable. For the same reason, men don't mind a hairy chest because it is considered masculine, but women do not want any visible hair growth on their chests. Neither sex readily acquiesces to hair loss or graying hair, and hats, caps, and cover-the-gray hair products are big business with the over-forty set.

Some people swear their hair turned gray almost overnight, but for most people, graying occurs by degrees. Experts say that the best way to slow down the graying of your hair is to relax. Although the tendency for hair to gray and the age and rate at which it does so is primarily determined by heredity and hormones, research indicates that stress contributes to graying hair too.

Diet also plays a role in hair health,

as it does in the quality of other body functions. The B vitamins, called "stress vitamins," have a calming effect on the nervous system. Because these vitamins become depleted when you are under stress, they are linked to hair growth and graying hair. A deficiency of zinc in the diet has been said to cause hair loss and baldness. Another associated cause of hair loss is crash dieting.

The wear and tear on your hair caused by the way you treat it also contributes to hair loss. One type of baldness referred to as traction alopecia is caused by too much pull on the hair. This condition is most often found in women who wear tight pony tails or braids or set their hair in tightly wound curlers. Hair can also be damaged by rough combing and vigorous brushing with overly stiff brushes.

Other hair damage and loss comes from harsh chemicals found in hair coloring and bleaching and perming solutions. Because hair is porous, it can absorb anything from air pollution to chemical solutions.

How Hair Grows

Let's take a closer look at how hair grows. Hair is present all over the body in some form, with the exception of the palms of the hands and the soles of the feet. It grows at a rate of about one inch per month. One of the most interesting hair characteristics is that even though all hair consists of the same chemical regardless of where it grows, the amount of hair growth and the length of time in which growth takes place varies tremendously from place to place. At any given time, hair in certain areas is in a growing phase, and in other are as it is in a resting phase. Eyebrows, for instance, never get longer than one inch. Once an eyebrow hair falls out, it takes a long time for one to grow back because the growing phase in the eyebrow area is very short, and the resting phase is very long.

Humans do not shed their hair like dogs and cats because the hair on these animals is always either in a growing or a resting phase. When the growing phase is over and the resting phase begins, a great deal of the hair on animals falls out or sheds. In humans, the growth and rest phases are occurring simultaneously, and hair is growing and falling out at the same time.

At any given time, approximately 70 percent of hair on the scalp is in the growing phase, and 30 percent is in the resting phase. Some of the hair in the resting phase will fall out during its natural cycle. This normal loss amounts to between 80 and 110 hairs a day. In order for the normal cycle to continue, hair must replace itself at the same rate it is falling out. There are many factors which can impact the ratio of these growth and rest phases.

The most common factor in women is the changing level of hormones, which occurs with pregnancy or when the body's own hormones are being manipulated with birth control pills. Both birth control pills and pregnancy raise the female hormone level which pushes the scalp hair into a high-growth phase. Many women have noticed that during pregnancy or while they are taking birth control pills, they have a fuller, healthier head of hair. When they stop taking birth control pills or for several months after pregnancy, there is significant hair loss. The reason is that hair reverts to its normal growth rate. It does take some time to reestablish normality, and probably 100 percent of the hair won't come back, but the majority of it usually does in time.

Another common ailment affecting about 3 percent of the U.S. population is referred to as alopecia areata, which means hair loss in a certain area (patches of hair fall out). Scalp and beard are the most common areas in which this occurs. Although there are cases of anemia and thyroid problems associated with this type of hair loss, most cases are linked to stress.

The best news about alopecia areata is that even though substantial amounts of hair in certain areas may be lost, the hair will grow back within a period of time — up to 18 months. As is the case with male pattern baldness (to be discussed next), the hair is asleep and not dead; therefore, regrowth can be stimulated. Interestingly though, when hair returns, it usually grows back white and then turns back to its natural color. Treatment is aimed at preventing further hair loss and speeding up the regrowth process. Treatment from a dermatologist may consist of cortisone creams and injections if necessary.

Male Pattern Baldness

This is the most common type of hair loss which affects men. Hair loss associated with male pattern baldness results from a combination of an inherited genetic trait and the male hormone testosterone. The male hormone acts on certain hair follicles and destroys them. A man can inherit the trait for male pattern baldness from either his mother or father. However, he can inherit it from his father only if his father is bald. His mother may carry the gene for baldness and pass it down to her son without ever losing any of her own hair. While about 15 percent of men of the European geographical race have male pattern baldness, the condition is less common among men from other genetic backgrounds.

There are a number of different patterns of this kind of baldness — loss of hair in the front, on both sides, from the crown of the scalp, from the central part of the scalp, from the entire head except over the ears, from the very back part of the scalp, from the entire head, and a combination of areas. Both the pattern of hair loss and the tendency for hair loss are inherited.

Although cases are rarer and not as noticeable as those associated with male pattern baldness, a number of women have a condition known as female pattern baldness. Typically, this kind of hair loss in women results in thinning hair but not total baldness. This condition is inherited and usually occurs after menopause.

Rogaine®

The drug Minoxidil has been used for many years to treat high blood pressure. In the process of lowering blood pressure, many patients who were taking the drug began to notice new hair on their scalp and face and thicker hair on their arms and legs. Doctors got the idea of using the drug to grow hair. Solutions were made from the tablet form to be applied to the skin. In testing situations, solutions were mixed and applied to the scalp in lotion or ointment form. In many instances, hair began to appear. Scientifically controlled studies began, and results showed that about 70 percent of the people who used this drug topically actually did begin to grow hair in the treated areas.

In the summer of 1988, Minoxidil was approved by the FDA and began to be marketed in the United States under the name Rogaine. It was the first drug to be approved for the purpose of growing hair. Rogaine appears to be effective on male as well as female pattern baldness. Its mechanism of action is unknown, and it has its drawbacks. First of all, it does not work on everyone. Quality control can be a problem depending on the source of the drug. The drug is quite expensive — about $50 a month — and results take a long time to show up. After two to four months, patients using Rogaine may begin to see new hair growth in the form of a very few fine hairs. Discontinuing the drug ensures the return of the original baldness pattern. Side effects seem primarily to be local skin irritations in some patients using the drug. From studies available so far, it appears that this treatment is more effective in people who have patchy balding problems rather than total alopecia.

So far, we have not found a way to cure or prevent baldness. Since hair loss and baldness are perceived as very undesirable conditions by so many people, many patients are willing to do whatever is necessary to reverse hair loss. Several methods are used to cover bald areas of the scalp. Many wear a hairpiece or toupé. There are surgical methods of hair transplanting in which a physician surgically removes plugs of the patient's scalp that contain growing hair. These plugs are then transplanted to the bald areas. However, please consult your doctor before spending money on products and treatments which promise a cure for baldness or promise a new head of hair.

Hair Transplants

Surgical procedures to correct baldness were rare until the late 1950s, when a New York dermatologist, Dr. Norman Orentreich, reported his success with grafting clusters of hair follicles in small pieces of scalp which were taken from the hairy sides of the scalp and put into the bald areas. Since then, this kind of surgery has flourished because techniques have been improved, and many doctors have come to specialize in hair-transplant surgery.

There are several different approaches to hair-transplant surgery, but the most common procedure involves a punch-grafting technique and is called the "free" graft of hair to a bald area from another hairy area of the scalp. The surgical procedure "frees" the hair and its root or follicle from one area and plants it in another area.

Another technique is referred to as the "flap-over" method, which was devised by Dr. Jose Jure of Argentina. This method uses hair-bearing skin flaps which remain attached to their donor site for blood supply in order to transfer larger areas of hair which replace bald areas. It has been used very successfully in patients who have sufficient areas of healthy hair in close proximity to the bald areas.

A third technique is called the "strip graft," which is used to reconstruct the hairline at the front of the scalp. In this procedure, a healthy, narrow strip of scalp is removed from the back of the head and transplanted to the place at the top of the forehead where the hairline should be. Once the hairline has been reestablished with this strip graft, other bald areas can be filled in with the best-suited hair-transplant method.

Hair Weaving

We do not recommend hair weaving because it has proven to be a medically unsatisfying procedure. The body tends to reject the implants of foreign hair woven into the scalp, and there has been a high rate of infection associated with hair weaving. The FDA has condemned the weaving of artificial hair into the scalp as unsafe and ineffective.

Unwanted Hair

What do you do when hair grows where it isn't supposed to grow? When unwanted hair appears on a woman's face, there may be a number of causes. A main cause is linked to changing hormone levels in the body. When the level of certain hormones in a woman's body changes, stimulation of the hair follicles occurs, producing more hair than normal. When a woman discontinues oral contraceptives or hormone-replacement therapy, excessive hair growth on the face may occur. In some cases, changes in hair growth may be temporary and growth patterns may revert. Unfortunately, in many cases once the hair follicle is stimulated, it does not revert to its old pace, and in many cases, reintroduction of birth control pills or hormone therapy does not slow down hair growth.

Many people have found electrolysis to be an effective method for removing unwanted hair. It is used on all parts of the face and the body — except the nose and ears — and works by directing a tiny, split-second impulse down to the root of the hair which destroys it so that the root will not produce another hair again. There is a slight tingling sensation involved, but it is not a painful procedure. There is usually some temporary redness after treatment, but healing after electrolysis is generally rapid, with no signs of the treatment remaining on the skin.

A very important consideration involved in electrolysis is the need for strict sterilization procedures performed by an experienced, licensed electrologist. The use of disposable needles is stressed in order to control communicable diseases.

Healthy Nails

Nails are made of hardened skin cells. The tissue below the nail from which the nails grow is called the matrix. Near the root of the nail the cells are smaller and carry less blood, and the white crescent-shaped area representing these cells is called the lunula (from luna, meaning moon).

If a nail is torn off, it can grow back again providing the matrix has not been too severely damaged. White spots on the nail are compared to bruises on the skin. These white spots will disappear as the nail grows out. The state of your general health can be reflected in nail growth. However, most diets of people in the United States today are sufficient to produce healthy nails.

The majority of problems with nail growth and nail health today are caused by harmful chemicals and treatments. Women who are concerned with nail fashion trends are abusing their nails more today than ever before. The widespread use of certain cosmetic nail applications is a perfect example of a mismatch between what may be considered attractive and what is healthy. When people glue their nails with harmful chemicals, apply false nails and subject their nails to acrylic processes which destroy the nail bed and weaken the entire nail structure, the result is very unhealthy nails.

If you don't believe it, find someone who has been applying false nails for a period of time and has decided to discontinue the practice and regrow their own nails. Ask them what their nails looked like when they removed the false nails and how long it took to restore their own nails to normal. Glues and products containing formaldehyde should never be used on the nails.

Eating a well-balanced diet and maintaining a healthy body is the best advice for keeping attractive, healthy nails. We recommend a very basic nail-care routine because in nail care, less is usually better.

Growing attractive, healthy nails is quite simple. Keep hands clean and pay particular attention to cleaning underneath nails. Cleanse gently. Be very careful not to probe beneath or around the cuticle with sharp metal or wooden sticks because this is where the new nail is formed. Trauma to the cuticle area causes nails to grow creased with lines. Do not cut or scrape in the cuticle area because this can cause pain and infection. Gently push cuticles back when you get out of the shower or bath, when they are soft and pliable. If excess cuticle grows onto the nail itself, this skin may be gently clipped. Do not break the skin at the cuticle. Keep nails filed smoothly with a fine emery board. Nails which are filed in a flatter and rounded shape do not break as easily as nails which are filed in a pointed shape. The less done to nails the better. There

is nothing wrong with nail polish that protects the nail. By establishing a nail style that is not too long, nails will stay consistently more attractive than nails grown to extreme lengths. It is tempting to replace a broken nail with a false one. One false nail leads to another. So if you are tempted to replace a broken nail with a false nail or glue the broken nail just until it grows back, remember that your nail will not grow back in a normal, healthy condition. It is best to allow the nail to grow back naturally — without exposure to harmful chemicals.

Younger-Looking Hands

People who have had cosmetic surgery and whose faces look younger than their age often want to know what can be done to produce younger-looking hands. Brown spots on hand skin are a telltale sign of aging and damage associated with sun exposure.

The first problem is a lack of a uniform color. The skin on the hands shows speckled and freckled skin characterized by what is referred to as "age spots" and "liver spots." The latter spots do not have anything to do with the liver. They usually have to do with sun exposure. They are actually superficial discolorations which are produced by concentrated folds of freckles. The tendency to have age or liver spots is inherited and accelerated by age and sun exposure.

131

These spots can be removed by freezing with liquid nitrogen and then using a bleaching agent applied to the areas during the healing process. Certain types of mild skin peels using glycolic or trichloracetic acids (but not phenol) are also effective if properly administered by a doctor experienced with this procedure. A peel is even more difficult to perform on the hands than it is on the face.

It is also possible to treat fine lines and wrinkles on the hands with injectable collagen which smooths out the surface of the skin and plumps up the creases. Like all injectable collagen treatments, this therapy is temporary and will have to be repeated in order to maintain the results. (See the "Soft-Tissue Augmentation" section for more information.)

Spider Veins

Some people are prone to developing tiny broken blood vessels on the face and other parts of the body. Commonly referred to as spider veins, the main type which occurs on the face and above the waist are the purplish, reddish veins called telangiectasias.

The primary cause is the ever-present destructive radiation from the sun. Exposure to sun causes skin to lose its natural collagen layer so that the network of tiny veins below the skin's surface can show through the thinned skin. Female hormones also play a part in producing this unsightly problem. That is why more women are bothered

by this problem than men. Spider veins tend to increase during pregnancy and during birth control pills and hormone-replacement therapy. Unfortunately, once the pregnancy is over or the hormone-related oral medications are discontinued, the spider veins which appeared do not usually disappear.

Another similar and equally annoying type of blood vessel problem appears on the face usually around the nose or the middle portions of the cheeks. These unsightly little vessels are also caused by changing hormone levels, sun damage, and the low-grade trauma brought on by tugging, pulling, and stretching the skin. This trauma can be aggravated by handling or treating skin harshly when cleansing or applying makeup.

Varicose Veins

Although many people complain about broken veins in the face, the most common area of complaint is the legs. In addition to broken vessels, other more serious vein problems, such as the bluish, swollen, cord-like veins referred to as varicose veins, are primarily problems in the legs. The culprit here is gravity and chronic elevated pressure in the veins. This weakens the walls of the veins, producing the dilated unsightly appearance.

More women complain about this problem than men. Many men share the problem, but it is covered up by hair or long pants. Unlike spider veins, which are mostly unsightly, varicose veins can be a painful problem. Some of the contributing causes are obesity, long hours of standing, and pregnancy. Although varicose veins are inherited, all of us are at risk as we get older, as our veins become less elastic and the supporting muscles and skin become weaker.

Varicose veins occur when the walls of the veins are weak or the valves in the veins which regulate the flow of blood back to the heart malfunction. The best advice is to watch for symptoms and to see your doctor early. Some of the signs of varicose veins in the early stages are bluish, swollen blood vessels. A common symptom is tired, aching feet and legs which feel unusually swollen and full. These symptoms traditionally occur after a long period of standing or sitting still. The symptoms get worse as the days go on, rather than disappearing quickly. Should you experience any of these symptoms, see a physician who specializes in the detection and treatment of varicose veins. If varicose veins are detected in the early stages, more serious symptoms and complications can be avoided.

Exercise plays an important role in prevention. Walking, cycling, jogging, and swimming work on legs and help prevent varicose veins by strengthening muscles and maintaining good blood flow. Eating a high-fiber diet rich in whole grains, bran, wheat germ, fresh fruits, and salads helps prevent varicose veins and keeps the condition from getting worse.

If you must stand or sit for long periods, remember to flex your leg muscles and move your toes around frequently to stimulate blood flow. When you sit, avoid crossing your legs. Do not wear items of clothing which bind at the waist or calf. These act like tourniquets. When you're at home, go barefoot; this strengthens the foot muscles and improves blood flow.

Treating Vein Problems

Treatments vary by type and location of the problem. The three major areas of concern are the face, breasts, and legs. At present, there are also three major treatment types: electric current, laser beams, and injection of various materials. On the face, where the tiny spider veins occur, the most effective treatment is to eradicate the vein with an electric needle. This treatment is rarely painful because the needle is so small and the electric current is very low, and in most cases no anesthesia is given. Generally, a spider vein on the face can be treated in a matter of seconds with good cosmetic results, and no aftercare is required. Recurrence happens about 25 percent of the time, but the treatment is inexpensive and basically painless and can be repeated as often as is required. Laser treatment can be used in the face, but it is generally more expensive and can be dangerous if performed by an inexperienced person. Injectable materials should never be used on the face because of scarring and possible harm to vital structures.

Treatment on the breast is generally limited to use of laser beams and electric needle. Laser treatment continues to be improved for the treatment of vascular problems, and not all doctors have the most advanced technology. This is an area where choosing the right doctor who is experienced in technique and who has the most up-to-date equipment is very crucial to obtaining the best results.

Sclerotherapy

Tiny veins and vessels on the legs are best treated by sclerotherapy. A concentrated solution of saline (salt water) or a substance called aethoxisclerol are injected into the vein. The solution causes the vein to shrink so that it can no longer carry blood. This rather simple procedure has been improved in recent years by the advent of tiny needles. These enable the doctor to enter the blood vessel easily and leak less of the injected material outside the blood vessel. Patients must wear a compression dressing for 72 hours after injection and avoid any vigorous exercise for three days.

There are some side effects associated with these injection treatments. The ankles may swell for several days, and patients may complain of feeling dehydrated. Brown spots can occur at the injection site but usually fade within several weeks. In rare situations in which the injected solution leaks out of the vessels, healing may leave a small scar. In even rarer cases, phlebitis may occur. It is very important to review your medical history with a doctor who is both qualified and experienced in treating vein problems. Specialists who frequently treat these problems are dermatologists, plastic surgeons, and vascular surgeons. Excellent treatment methods are available to improve many conditions which may not be life threatening but which certainly affect how you perceive yourself and are perceived by others.

The next section explains the many wonderful options in cosmetic surgery including those that improve on the work of nature and those that turn back the hands of time.

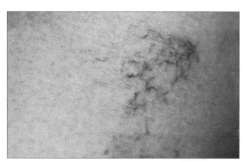

Before sclerotherapy to improve spider veins on the leg

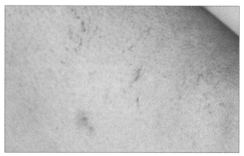

After sclerotherapy to improve spider veins on the leg

The New Age of Cosmetic Surgery

With all best efforts to take good care of your body and your skin, there will inevitably be the day when each of us looks in the mirror and sees the dreaded first signs of aging: wrinkled or sagging skin. As we get older, nothing stays quite the same.

Until recently we had only our best preventive methods and cosmetic products to help us defend against and camouflage the march of time. We could do our best, but eventually we just had to accept an aging appearance as a fact of life.

Today, we live in a new age of advanced and improved medical options. We have resources and capabilities which were unheard of in previous generations. Tremendous progress has been made in cosmetic surgery, offering good news for the millions of people who find themselves looking older and who want to improve their appearance. At last, the capabilities of cosmetic surgery and society's acceptance of self-improvement are coming of age together.

In many ways, society's growing acceptance of cosmetic surgery is due to today's widespread communications network. Through television, radio, and the print world of magazines and newspapers, we have developed a closer, more intimate knowledge of each other. As communications have increased, we have expanded our scope. Doors have opened to new opportunities and knowledge. The chance to excel, to improve, to learn, and to grow also have come into focus as we share information and resources. The media's positive attention to all forms of healthy self-improvement and society's enthusiastic embrace of research and practical applications that lead to healthy bodies and minds have done wonders for cosmetic surgery too.

Gone are the days when people were secretive about fixing a problem or taking a few years off their faces and bodies. We are no longer made to feel embarrassed about wanting to look our best or about making positive changes. We no longer have to learn to live with physical features we do not like or accept the unattractive signs of aging as unalterable facts of life. An attractive appearance is something we want for ourselves and look for in each other, and today it is not only possible to improve appearance, it is widely accepted to do so.

This new acceptance level applies equally to how we see ourselves and those around us. We are far more tolerant of and even happy about our individual differences, but we are far more demanding in our efforts to achieve our own goals and succeed in life the way we want to. We are also far more receptive to applying the resources of modern technology and human knowledge to help us match the image we have of ourselves on the inside with the appearance we present to the world. After all, most people have a beautiful, youthful spirit, and cosmetic surgery can help keep it that way.

BLENDING ART AND SCIENCE

Have you ever wondered about our sense of beauty? Why do we perceive certain people to be attractive and others unattractive? How and why do we classify beauty, and where does the need to do so come from? If beauty is, in fact, a matter of millimeters in one direction or the other, is beauty an art, or is it a science? Perhaps it is a combination of the two.

According to scientists, every human brain functions as a classifying machine. The ability to classify began as a matter of survival when early man had to know every detail of the world around him. He made a science of evaluating and classifying all aspects of his surroundings and learning how each element compared to others. This way, when he needed to know something or when an emergency occurred, the knowledge of his environment was there to serve and protect him.

As a vital part of survival, human beings evolved to become great masters of observation with highly sensitive powers to discern between many things. What could they use? What did they like? What did they want to avoid? What brought pleasure? The way in which we distinguish and classify today came from

our early ancestors' basic need to distinguish between all things within their environment, as did the creation of art and the appreciation of beauty.

People continued to classify even after the need was not vitally linked to food, shelter, and protection. Indeed, this trait — classifying information, making comparisons, responding to what is visually appealing — is a deeply rooted part of human nature. We continue this practice today — from collecting rare antiques and art objects to watching and appreciating members of the opposite sex on the beach.

Aesthetics

The word *aesthetic* means appreciating beauty. Desmond Morris, author of many wonderful books including *Intimate Behavior* and *Manwatching*, refers to "aesthetic behavior" as the reaction people have to what is beautiful in both art and nature. Morris points out that our pursuit of beauty is difficult to explain; it isn't directly related to survival, but we can't ignore it either.

According to Morris, who has spent a lifetime observing and studying human and animal behavior, "Any objective survey of how people spend their time must include many hours of beauty-reaction. There is no other way to describe the response of men and women who can be found standing silently in front of paintings in an art gallery, or sitting quietly listening to music, or watching dancing, or viewing sculpture, or gazing at flowers, or wandering through landscapes, or savouring wines. The advanced winetaster even goes so far as to spit out the wine after tasting it, as if to underline that it is his need for beauty that is being quenched and not his thirst."

Reactions to Beauty

The "beauty-reaction" is both cultural and individual. There is no standard of beauty that has remained fixed through-out the ages, and from one part of the globe to another, the idea of what is beautiful — both in the arts and in the human form — varies immensely. In *Manwatching*, a study of the behavior of homosapiens, Morris takes us on a tour of beauty contestants throughout the ages, describing the vital statistics of some of history's rarest beauty queens.

"The only measurements quoted for the current Miss World contestants are their so-called vital statistics — their bust, waist, and hip measurements. The average in inches for a typical contest works out to be at 35-24-35. If we turn back the clock to prehistoric times we cannot compare these figures with the real females of the past, but if we assume that the carved figurines of ancient females that have survived represent the ideal of those earlier times, then some startling differences emerge. One of the earliest of all 'beauty queens' is the Venus of Willendorf, a small stone carving from central Europe. If we consider her Miss Stone Age of 20,000 B.C., then, had she lived, her vital statistics would have been 96-89-96. Moving forward to 2000 B.C., Miss Indus Valley would have measured 45-34-63, and in the Late Bronze Age, Miss Cyprus of 1500 B.C. would have registered 43-42-44. Later still, Miss Amlash of 1000 B.C. would have offered the startling proportions of 38-44-78, but Miss Syria of 1000 B.C., only a short distance away, would have measured an almost modern 31-26-36."

While what is perceived as attractive may vary greatly, the need to classify is very strong in all people. Human beings are unique in the animal world in that, to a large extent, we choose our mates according to what is visually attractive. However, modern-day psychologists warn us of the potential dangers in picking a mate for reasons of mere physical attraction. Many relationships fail when partners realize that, as individuals, they have little in common to bond them together. Thus, many people in the 1990s are putting more emphasis on being well rounded, by developing a healthy body and mind as well as physical attractiveness.

Even so, the basic human response to beauty — as it is perceived on an individual, gender, and cultural basis — is just as strong today as it ever was. And as long as we allow plenty of room for individual differences, the "beauty-reaction" can be a very positive part of modern living.

We are who we are, and an important function of the modern-day classification process involves finding out about ourselves and learning — as our ancient ancestors did — all about the world around us. From the many ways in which we create art from nature, to the many ways modern technology allows us to improve on nature, we are judged by how creative we are and by how we employ the beauty within ourselves and in the world around us. As Morris concludes, "It is the game that the human animal plays with consummate skill."

Variations on a Theme

We live in a time when men and women are their own role models and believe in making the most of themselves as individuals. We define our looks, our style, our fashion, for example, as well as our career and lifestyle goals. An amazing number of choices and options are well within our reach: the potential for higher education, greater health and longevity, diverse careers, happiness, and an attractive appearance. There are scientists, teachers, writers, and doctors who have devoted their professional lives to expanding human potential. We have created an age of information which no doubt evolved from the human need to classify, and the worldwide advancements have brought options unheard of in any other time.

Though often taken for granted, the opportunities to be our best and look our best in every way are distinct modern phenomena. Like the science of understanding what creates health and fitness in the human body, the science of developing an attractive appearance and image is now within our reach. We have the modern choices of understanding what our options are for improvement and classifying what best meets our individual needs.

Plastic Surgery: Art through Science

No discussion of the subject of personal improvements would be complete without an in-depth look at plastic surgery. As a medical specialty, plastic surgery has evolved to include a broad spectrum of medical advances. Yet many people do not really understand what these options are, or if plastic surgery is truly a viable option. This section will take a good look at all the various procedures within the specialty and help you classify for yourself. Many people have already developed an opinion about plastic surgery, or so they think. Either they say "I'm very interested" or "That's not for me." But others become interested in plastic surgery only when they learn more about it.

Some people know they want to have plastic surgery in order to improve a certain physical feature or to bring their appearance in line with their self-image. Many of these consider plastic surgery to be an important part of how they will "age gracefully." People who have had a good result from a plastic surgery procedure are the specialty's greatest proponents. They have first-hand knowledge of how making an improvement in their appearance opened up doors of potential for them.

Plastic surgery is a hybrid of art and science. It is medical science's response to enhancing the human form and improving on nature. For reconstructing birth defects and repairing injuries, it is modern science at its best. But plastic surgery can also go beyond physical healing; in many cases it helps transform a person's self-image by simply refining or improving a physical feature.

If you ever have the chance to know any plastic surgeons personally, you will find that many of them are very artistic in nature. A surprising number of plastic surgeons paint, sculpt, write poetry, make jewelry, and pursue other art forms. Plastic surgeons have vivid "beauty-reactions," a quality which many think leads them to specialize in creating beauty in the human form through medical science.

Like an architect, who is challenged to build a building that will stand the test of time in efficiency and design, the plastic surgeon is concerned with both function and form. Again, as an architect would consider the terrain of the building site as well as the purpose and use of the building, the plastic surgeon takes care to consider the individual's potential, the expectations involved, and the health and well-being of the patient.

Self-Enhancement with Cosmetic Surgery

Many people ask where the word *plastic* in plastic surgery comes from. It comes from the Greek word *plastikos*, which means to mold or give form. Molding and giving form to the human body is what plastic surgery is all about.

Generally speaking, there are two specialties within plastic surgery. Reconstructive surgery restores or improves physical form and function and minimizes disfigurements from birth defects, accidents, and disease. Aesthetic or cosmetic surgery, which is one of the fastest-growing medical specialties of our time, improves the appearance of facial and body features. Both specialties within plastic surgery offer people tremendous improvements in the quality of their lives by enhancing both their form and function.

Candidates for Plastic Surgery

There is little doubt as to who the candidates are for reconstructive surgery. People of all ages have special problems which generally require immediate attention. It is wonderful that medicine has many ways of correcting physical problems and defects which result from injury, accidents, disease, and birth defects. In reconstructive surgery, patients and their families are concerned with fixing problems that cause physical as well as emotional trauma.

The candidates for cosmetic surgery are individuals who recognize a specific area in their appearance which could be improved and who have a personal desire to make a change. A person, for example, may want to improve an unattractive physical feature, bring one feature into balance with others, or stay younger looking longer. The decision to have cosmetic surgery may not be essential to physical health, but it can certainly make a significant contribution to the individual's overall well-being. Most cosmetic surgery is elective, a matter of personal choice. We live in a time where modern medicine has advanced past the point of responding only to our critical needs and is now able to turn some of its attention to our elective needs and desires. These medical options are increasing in number not only in plastic surgery but also in other medical fields.

Life today has evolved to a point where we are not so much concerned with physical survival as we are with the quality of survival. This "ultimate modern convenience" is reflected in every aspect of the way we manage our lifestyles and careers. Interestingly, we don't take it for granted. We are willing to work hard to achieve a higher quality of life, with each generation trying to improve on the previous one's effort. For most of us, the pursuit of higher quality is the greatest personal achievement, and — like other forms of science which have made life easier and more efficient — medicine has followed suit.

In essence, art and science have come together very successfully in cosmetic surgery. And since we human beings have proven to be aesthetic creatures who naturally relate to personal appearances and gravitate toward beauty in the world around us, cosmetic surgery is proving to be a very positive part of many lives.

The Decision to Have Plastic Surgery

Many people think about possibly having cosmetic surgery, but the only way to find out what's involved and if it is a viable option for you is to have a consultation visit with a cosmetic surgeon.

Most plastic surgeons charge only a nominal fee for an initial consultation. The first step is to select a qualified, experienced plastic surgeon and call for an appointment. (See the next section, "Choosing a Plastic Surgeon.") Ask to set up a consultation visit, as you are in the fact-finding stage. You will have an appointment, and the educational process can begin.

If, on the first visit, you want only to get information and talk to the doctor, explain this to the staff member who schedules your appointment. It is a good idea to ask for written information about the practice and the cosmetic procedure which interests you. These materials can be sent in the mail, and you can have a chance to review them and prepare some questions before your visit with the doctor. Many plastic surgeons have nurses and physician's assistants, who specialize in patient education. They can be excellent information resources and are well trained to answer many of your questions.

In the next several sections we will review some background information about plastic surgeons and their surgical facilities. It may not make for the most interesting reading, but anyone considering plastic surgery needs to know this information. After the short homework course, we'll get right into discussing the more exciting information about the many different face and body procedures available in cosmetic surgery.

Choosing a Plastic Surgeon

Before you explore the possibilities of cosmetic surgery, please understand that the results of plastic surgery depend on the surgeon's training, experience, and ability to perform the specific procedure. Learning how to choose a plastic surgeon is the very first step.

The specialized training to become a plastic surgeon takes many years. First, four years of undergraduate college are required, then four years of medical school, an approved surgery residency of at least three years, and a plastic surgery residency of another two to three years.

Upon completion of this extensive curriculum, the doctor can obtain certification by the American Board of Plastic Surgery only after passing rigorous written and oral examinations administered by extensively trained and experienced plastic surgeons.

The American Board of Medical Specialties (ABMS) exists to promote high standards in patient care through the establishment of criteria for physician training. Its associate members include six of the major organizations within the medical community, including the American Medical Association. The ABMS recognizes one certifying board per specialty, each of which tests and certifies physicians in their field of expertise. The ABMS has designated the American Board of Plastic Surgery as the only one of its member boards to certify in the specialty of plastic surgery. There is no separate ABMS-recognized certifying board for cosmetic surgery.

Do not be confused by other official-sounding boards and certifications; in most U.S. states it is legal for any physician who holds a medical license, with or without surgical training, to call him or herself a plastic or cosmetic surgeon.

Because choosing the right surgeon is the single most important factor in the success of cosmetic or reconstructive surgery, be careful in your selection. Get more than one opinion. Verify the surgeon's training and experience thoroughly. Plastic surgery is a very sophisticated medical specialty, and it takes many years and technique-dependent training to be able to do good work and get good results.

When you visit with a plastic surgeon, talk candidly about your expectations, and feel free to ask questions. Tell the doctor about yourself and the reason for your visit. Ask to see before-and-after photographs of the doctor's patients, and find out how often the doctor has performed the procedure you desire. Only after you have established mutual objectives and a feeling of compatibility with a plastic surgeon who has the appropriate credentials should you move ahead with the decision to have cosmetic surgery.

If you have any questions about a plastic surgeon's board certification or how to locate a qualified plastic surgeon in your community, you can consult the *ABMS Compendium of Certified Medical Specialists* or *The Directory of Medical Specialists*, available at most libraries.

Physicians certified by the American Board of Plastic Surgery are eligible for membership in the American Society of Plastic and Reconstructive Surgeons (ASPRS) and the American Society for Aesthetic Plastic Surgery (ASAPS). The ASPRS represents the full scope of plastic surgery: both reconstructive and cosmetic. ASAPS membership represents plastic surgeons who choose to concentrate their practices in cosmetic surgery. Both societies require comparable board certifications.

Anyone wanting to obtain a list of board-certified plastic surgeons specializing in aesthetic (cosmetic) surgery may call 1-800-635-0635 and ask for referral from the American Society for Aesthetic Plastic Surgery.

Your First Visit

The first visit to a plastic surgeon, like your first visit to any doctor, is called a consultation. Ideally, this will be a time when you learn answers to questions and find out about the cosmetic procedure or procedures which interest you. It is important to get written information such as brochures and pamphlets about cosmetic surgery procedures, the doctor's training and credentials, insurance (if applicable) and financial facts, and pre- and post-operative information about the surgery you desire. Take this written information home and read it carefully when you have plenty of quiet time. Be sure to understand what to expect before, during, and after surgery; learn how long it takes to return to normal after surgery; and write down any questions which need to be answered by the doctor. Keep in mind that a good doctor wants to hear your questions; by addressing them, the two of you are communicating about mutual expectations and realistic results. The doctor may also have instructional videos to show you, and this is an appropriate time to ask to see patients' before-and-after photographs. Be sure that the photographs you see represent the doctor's own work and not that of someone else.

During this visit, the doctor will examine you and take a medical history. You probably will have photographs taken because plastic surgeons use photography as a means to discuss your individual case, to explain what they want to do, and to document the before-and-after results. It is much easier for doctor and patient to communicate ideas when both are looking at the same picture. The purpose of the in-office photography is not to get a glamour shot but to capture the face and body from various angles and at certain profiles.

Sometimes patients bring photographs or magazine pictures of other people to the consultation in order to show the doctor how they want their nose, face, or other feature to look after cosmetic surgery has been performed. Please keep in mind that these types of requests are not realistic because the pictures are of other people, not you. The realistic results cosmetic surgery can accomplish include bringing the features of your face into balance and proportion with each other. Your nose needs to match your face. The reshaping of a certain facial feature or the recontouring of your body is a totally individual process.

A hair stylist once explained that when a client brings in a picture of a particular hair style and asks him to duplicate it on her, he usually has to say, "That will be very difficult because your hair needs to be cut and styled according to its own texture and weight. It also needs to be cut and styled to compliment your face. It's next to impossible to force your hair to do something it's not made to do. Besides, it's so much better to have your own style anyway."

The same idea applies to cosmetic surgery because there are many individual components to be considered. Many doctors use visual-imaging systems which are computer systems designed to help the doctor and patient communicate about the projected results. With these systems, an actual video image of the patient is projected onto a monitor screen. The doctor uses a computerized drawing technique to shape, shade, and draw the patient's after-surgery image. This new image is projected onto the screen right next to the patient's actual unretouched image.

Video imaging represents an effective communications tool, but keep in mind that what you see on the computer screen is a two-dimensional image, and your face and body are three-dimensional. You cannot take the computer image literally. Plus, many people who are trained to draw on the computer system can create a visual image, but the actual surgical result depends on the ability and experience of the plastic surgeon who performs the operation. (See section called "Computer Imaging.")

Whether the doctor uses a video-imaging system, photographs, or drawings, be sure that you have thoroughly discussed your expectations of surgery and that they are in line with the results the surgery can realistically provide. Cosmetic surgery can improve and enhance your appearance and boost your self-esteem, but it does not change your life and your relationships for you. That part is up to you.

Anesthesia

Improved methods of anesthesia have allowed great advancements in surgical procedures during recent years. Because of the improvements and reduced side effects, all types of surgery are easier on the patient and recovery time is shortened. Surgeons can perform the operation more quickly, which cuts down on the trauma and speeds up the healing process.

In elective cosmetic surgery cases, most procedures are performed under local anesthesia with intravenous sedation. Patients rarely remember anything about the surgery and do not feel any pain. In cases where extensive surgery or multiple procedures require it, general anesthesia will be used. General anesthesia used during cosmetic surgery of the face is not the same as deep anesthesia which is given during operations of the stomach, lungs, heart, or other organs.

Before surgery, the surgeon will discuss any anesthesia options and requirements in detail. Patients will be given written instructions in advance of surgery. It is very important that patients follow these instructions exactly during the days or weeks before and after surgery in order to protect their health and more nearly ensure the surgical results.

Combining Cosmetic Surgery Procedures

Improved surgical techniques and anesthesia have facilitated the option of having more than one cosmetic surgery procedure performed at a time. Also, patients who are scheduled for other types of medically necessary surgery are frequently choosing to have cosmetic surgery performed at the same time. The advantages of multiple procedures are reduced costs and only one recovery period.

The safety of combining surgeries is enhanced by administering high levels of intravenous fluids and by the use of antibiotics. Safety also depends on keeping the total operating time under five hours. It is possible for an experienced plastic surgeon to complete facelift, eyelid, chin-implant, and nasal surgeries; tummy tuck and liposuction; or fat suctioning on several areas of the body within this time frame. If multiple procedures are to be performed at once, generally face and neck procedures are done at one time and body contouring at another.

The decision to combine surgical procedures — whether they are elective or medically necessary operations — depends on the types of surgeries, the patient's health, and the surgeon or surgeons' skill and experience levels.

Informed Consent

Cosmetic surgery, like all other surgery, is not an exact, risk-free science. Therefore, it is the doctor's responsibility to provide detailed information about the risk-management side of plastic surgery and anesthesia, as well as manufacturers' information explaining all aspects of any implant devices which may be incorporated into the surgery. Although significant complications are rare in the hands of experienced surgeons, doctors will have you read and sign that you are aware of the possibilities of complications. Feel free to ask your doctor any questions you have about informed-consent documents, whose language unfortunately can get rather technical.

Informed-consent documents are a part of this country's medical system and are required by insurance companies as well. Do not be frightened by them because the information is designed to protect you. Just be sure you talk to your doctor and get your "plain-talk" questions answered in detail.

An important part of the patient's responsibility is to understand any possible risks or complications which can occur in cosmetic surgery procedures or as a result of anesthesia. Although complications are very rare, it is necessary for each person deciding to have cosmetic surgery to consider all aspects of risk management. The best patient is informed and educated, asks plenty of questions, and gets all the answers.

Scars from Cosmetic Surgery

Patients always ask, "Will there be scars?" The answer is, anytime there is a procedure involving any type of incision, there will be varying degrees of scarring. The extent to which scarring occurs depends on the extent of the incision made and the genetically determined degree to which each individual's skin scars. People with dark skin and olive complexions and Orientals tend to scar more than people with fair skin or light complexions. Sun exposure increases the amount of scarring, as does smoking. The good news is that plastic surgeons are trained to make incisions which are as small as possible and, whenever possible, concealed in natural skin folds. Even scars which are very red in color and are very noticeable at first will, in the course of a couple of years, begin to fade and become less noticeable.

Smoking and Cosmetic Surgery

If you decide to have cosmetic surgery, it is generally advised not to smoke, use other tobacco products, or chew nicorette gum for two weeks before and after surgery. Aside from the obvious health risks associated with tobacco and smoking, surgeons ask patients to adhere to this abstinence policy very strictly because nicotine from the tobacco constricts blood vessels and reduces blood flow. Smoking produces carbon monoxide, which is absorbed into the body through the lungs.

Surgical procedures involving elevation of tissues — such as facelift, eyelid surgery, and tummy tuck — require the blood supply to the skin be partially and temporarily interrupted. These delicate areas are dependent on a limited blood supply during the time of surgery when the tissues are elevated and afterwards during healing. If the blood vessels which supply oxygenated blood to these tissues are constricted due to the residual effects of nicotine, and if the oxygen supply is reduced due to the effects of carbon monoxide (which is poisonous to the tissues), then the oxygen supply necessary to preserve healthy tissue is insufficient. As a result, the chances for scarring are greatly increased.

Also, like sun exposure, smoking will decrease the positive results obtained by cosmetic surgery because it speeds up the aging process, destroys the quality of skin tone, and causes wrinkles and creases all over the body. (See the section "Smoking and Second-Hand Smoke Health Risks.")

Video-Imaging Systems

One of the most important success factors in cosmetic surgery is patient-doctor communications. What the

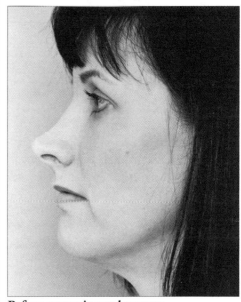

Before cosmetic nasal surgery

patient expects from the results of cosmetic surgery and what the doctor realistically can accomplish must be clearly established up front.

For many years, cosmetic surgeons used drawings as the best pictorial means of projecting after-surgery results. In many cases, the surgeon took a photograph of the patient before surgery and made a composite drawing from the photograph of how the face or body would look after the surgery was completed and healing had occurred. Naturally, this communications technique is dependent on the surgeon's artistic ability to draw and restricted by the limitations of the sketching medium itself. As anyone who has ever had a portrait drawn or painted knows, there is much room for individual interpretation. What you see in yourself and what the

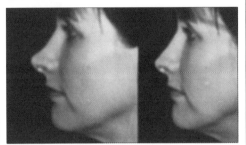
Patient shown on video-imaging computer: (left) before   (right) after imaging

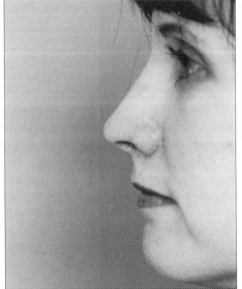
Patient shown after cosmetic nasal surgery has been performed

artist captures are often far apart.

Many people who evaluate the possibilities of cosmetic surgery say that the hardest part of the decision-making process is not being sure of how they will look afterwards. There are many variables involved, making the results of cosmetic surgery as individual as the people themselves. No matter how many before-and-after photographs you see of other patients who have had the same cosmetic surgery performed by the same doctor, there is much left to the imagination when your own face or body is involved.

The advent of computer-imaging systems is making a very positive difference in the decision-making process for cosmetic surgery because, properly used, this technology offers a better way to individualize and demonstrate the realistic opportunities for self-improvement. In the last several years, there have been extensive clinical evaluations of the hardware and software that form the basis of computer imaging systems. Medical experts and computer technologists have combined forces to study imaging technology for its practicality and effectiveness and have concluded that, *in the right hands*, these systems can increase communications by closing the gap between what the patient wants and what the doctor can do. They have also been shown to help decrease the trepidation the patient may feel as a result of the "unknown" factor in cosmetic surgery, help patients better understand and analyze their own appearances and the surgical options available, and increase the patient's post-surgical satisfaction.

Recent high-tech advances have made today's state-of-the-art imaging systems easier to use and more flexible in the doctor's ability to show detailed changes. Let's see how it works.

If a patient wants to have nose surgery to reshape the nose, the doctor first takes the patient's picture with an electronic video camera from a side-angle profile or a full-face front view. The image of the face is then digitized and recorded in high-resolution color and projected onto a large computer screen that looks just like a television. The actual image is projected onto one-half of the screen while a second copy of the image is projected onto the other side of the screen. The system's software provides electronic drawing capability which enables the doctor to make changes on the screen using trimming, blending, scaling, tapering, and shading techniques which reshape the nose and reflect how it will look after the surgery has been performed. The "before" image appears next to the "after" image on the screen so that the patient and doctor can discuss their expectations interactively using the images as visual references.

It is important to point out that, although the technical advantages of computer-imaging systems provide excellent tools for communications and teaching, the realistic results of any cosmetic surgery are only as good as the surgical skill and experience of the surgeon. Cosmetic surgery is not an exact science and its results represent improvement and not perfection. It is, however, safe to say that a picture is worth a thousand words and that computer-imaging technology represents an important advancement in how patients view themselves and how surgeons interpret the self-improvement cosmetic surgery options.

Cosmetic Surgery for Men

Although most cosmetic surgery is performed on women, the number of men who seek cosmetic surgery is definitely on the rise. According to statistics published by the American Society of Plastic and Reconstructive Surgeons, the number of men who had cosmetic surgery between 1984 and 1988 increased 69 percent. Of all cosmetic surgery patients in 1988, 16 percent of them were men versus 12 percent in 1984. The top choices for men ranked accordingly: nose surgery, eyelid surgery, liposuction or fat-suction surgery, and facelift surgery.

Cosmetic surgery has risen in popularity among men because more men are aware of the connection between appearance and personal and career successes. Plus, in these days and times, there is less stigma associated with cosmetic surgery for either sex; men no longer perceive it as an option for the rich and famous or as a vain luxury reserved for women. The number of procedures performed on men has also increased because the advances in surgical techniques yield more natural-looking results, which is what men, as well as women, are looking for. Also, today there is less downtime and out-of-work time involved.

Industry experts predict that the increasing numbers of men who have cosmetic surgery will continue to grow as more health-conscious men want to look as young as they feel. Recent studies point to the fact that men's motives for improving their appearances are closely linked to career. According to a survey of 375 managers at the Rochester Institute of Technology (RIT), 22 percent of the men agreed with the statement "I use my personal appearance to my advantage in getting things accomplished on the job." Interestingly, only 14 percent of women surveyed agreed with the same statement.

The Collagen Corporation Commission for the Study of Beauty and Aging recently sponsored a nationwide survey on the importance of appearance and job success. Key results from their survey support the RIT findings.

• 84 percent of men believed physical attractiveness is important for power and success on the job.

• 32 percent of men agreed that if they had a more youthful appearance, it would positively impact their job success.

• 42 percent of men felt that improving one thing about their face would help their career. The top priorities were nose, skin, hair, and eyelids.

In addition to the top-ranked procedures popular with men, others include collagen injections, derma-brasion, and chemical peel, which improve wrinkles, lines, creases, and scars; ear pinning to correct protruding ears; chin augmentation to enhance a weak-looking or recessed chin; and gynecomastectomy, which involves removal of excess or fatty tissue in the breast or chest area where many men tend to deposit fat.

Perhaps the most interesting part of the growing acceptance of cosmetic surgery by men is that their wives and female friends are overwhelmingly supportive. As one woman put it, "Any way you look at it, if we both look good, we both benefit. The pride we have in each other is increased, and any competition or jealousy we may feel as individuals is equalized."

Hospital Versus Surgicenter

A qualified plastic surgeon is usually on the staff of one or more accredited hospitals where surgery can be performed and where patients can stay overnight during the recovery period. In recent years, doctors have perfected surgical techniques and anesthesia procedures to such an extent that today, cosmetic surgery rarely requires a traditional extended hospital stay. Throughout the country, cosmetic surgeons perform many surgical procedures in a surgicenter, out-patient, or ambulatory clinic. Many plastic surgeons have their own freestanding surgicenters or surgical suites outside a hospital setting.

In out-patient surgery cases, the patient is often released after surgery to go home to be cared for by family, close friends, or in some cases a private nurse. Many cities have post-surgical care facilities where patients can recuperate after surgery when a hospital stay is not required. You may ask your doctor to recommend a post-surgical care center as a comfortable alternative to home care.

The main reason for the increased popularity of out-patient surgery with both surgeons and patients is that it minimizes the time and cost involved. The atmosphere in a surgicenter is usually very private, convenient, and less intimidating than a hospital and is there-fore more relaxing for a patient who is having elective surgery and is not sick.

There are regulations governing surgicenters, and some insurance companies have certain requirements which must be met in order to provide applicable coverage for procedures and services at the surgicenters. Well-respected, independent certifying groups such as the American Association of Accreditation of Ambulatory Plastic Surgery Facilities have set stringent standards for surgicenters and ambulatory clinics. They conduct on-site inspections and require that the facility be equipped with state-of-the-art equipment and meet safety precautions prior to certification.

Surgicenters should be equipped with standard safety equipment, monitoring devices, operating and recovery rooms and a qualified staff trained to handle any emergency. Equipment should include EKG and pulse monitors, anesthesia equipment, resuscitation equipment, and oxygen and emergency power sources. Surgicenters also must have access to a proper blood bank and a working agreement with a hospital close by should an emergency situation occur. A surgicenter must meet all state requirements and ideally has been certified by an independent organization such as the American Association of Ambulatory Plastic Surgery Facilities. If you have questions about an out-patient surgery facility, contact the local county, city, or state medical association in your area for more information.

The next sections provide information on cosmetic surgery and are arranged by procedure. They are divided into two main sections — procedures of the face and procedures of the body — and an overview introduces each group. It is probably a good idea to read all the information to get a general idea of what cosmetic surgery is about and what the options are. However, if you are specifically interested in one procedure, you'll probably want to move to that section first and read the others later. Throughout the various sections, you will find personal stories based on patients' experiences which offer special insights into how different people feel before, during, and after cosmetic surgery.

Cosmetic Surgery of the Face

People of all ages make connections by looking into each other's faces. We form our impressions of each other from facial expressions and facial gestures. We stare into each other's eyes and very often, words and other actions are unnecessary to express intention, desire, and other strong emotions. In conversation, from the moment our eyes meet, we begin to make ourselves known to each other. In a matter of seconds, we scan the entire face and features of another person, but we tend to concentrate on the most expressive features on the face — the eyes and mouth.

During social encounters, the attraction we feel for each other is commonly expressed by the way we look into each other's eyes. We express a wide range of emotions — love, humor, understanding, compassion, anger, fear — simply through the facial expressions we share.

Much has been written about the psychology of self-esteem, and experts agree that it is greatly influenced by how each of us relates to our own face. Cosmetic surgery has done wonders for someone who was born with an unattractive facial feature and for those whose facial features grow unattractive with age. From childhood to maturity, the way our faces are shaped, the size and angles of our facial features, and the balance and proportion of our facial contours and profiles play an important part in shaping the image we have of ourselves.

Psychology Today recently reported that 60 million Americans do not like their noses, 30 million do not like their chins, 6 million do not like their eyes, and another 6 million do not like their ears. Well, this year alone over 1 million of them will do something about it, and in the process of improving the features they do not like, they will also enhance the way they feel about themselves.

The Facelift, or Rhytidectomy

This section on facelift surgery is woven in between real stories told by patients who have had firsthand experience. These stories offer personal insight into some of the motivating factors behind their decisions, how they feel before and after, and what it's like to see the results.

Ruth (Age 64)

For the last 43 years, my husband Ben and I have had a wonderful marriage. We had so many good times and raised three beautiful daughters. About six years ago, Ben got sick and before he died last spring, he was an invalid who required my constant care. I wanted to care for Ben, and it was a labor of love, but anyone who has been through a similar situation knows how personally limiting it is. Ben is gone now, and I miss him more than words can express. Now I have to begin to live my life again as he would have wanted me to.

Shortly before Ben got sick, I had seen a plastic surgeon about a facelift, which is something I really wanted to do. Ben was supportive, but after he got sick it was impossible to think of. I put the idea out of my mind — but not completely — because I decided to have the facelift in September of this year. I wanted to have plenty of time to get myself together by Thanksgiving when all my children and grandchildren were coming to visit. I decided I probably needed to have my head examined before inviting them all at once, but I love to cook, and I couldn't wait to see my daughters' reactions to my new look.

At first, I thought I might be too old to think about cosmetic surgery, but my doctor assured me that I was not. I had been feeling like such a shut-in, and I had gotten to the point I didn't want to see myself in the mirror. The skin on my face and neck sagged, and I always looked tired. I had bags under my eyes and a lot of excess skin under my chin. I know I'm painting a pretty grim picture of myself, but every time I looked in the mirror I felt tired just seeing my face. I felt good and wanted to get out and live a full life again.

I actually ended up having more than one procedure because as my doctor explained, that was what I needed to accomplish the results I wanted. I had a facelift, as well as upper and lower eyelids, and while I was at it, I had my nose reshaped a little bit too. My doctor told me that reshaping my nose would make it look more in balance with my face once it was recontoured.

All I can say is that I have no regrets. All in all, the time involved from the day of the surgery until I felt like going out again was about two and a half weeks. I had quite a lot of bruising at first, but I really didn't have much pain at all. I was mostly tired and uncomfortable, but after the first week, every day seemed to get better and better.

As I write this story, my family has come and gone for Thanksgiving. When my daughters first saw me, they were thrilled. They just kept saying things like, "Mom, you look terrific." They were all very happy for me. Most of all I'm happy for myself because this has given me a new outlook. The past few years have been very hard, but I think this surgery will motivate me to get back out in the world again. At least now, I actually like seeing myself in the mirror again.

The facelift is a surgical procedure designed to reduce sagging skin on the face and neck, remove fatty tissue, and recontour the facial profile. As we discussed in the section "How Skin Ages," years of gravity pulling on the face cause it to become loose and saggy. Skin, muscles, and fatty tissue are not always attached directly to the bone, and the force of gravity causes a downward shift. The elastic quality of skin can be significantly reduced by sun exposure, smoking, and losing and regaining weight over the years. As these conditions occur, the defined facial contours associated with a youthful face tend to disappear. The loss of contour and skin tone and the change in the elasticity of the skin are what cause the appearance of the face to change with time.

The facelift procedure is not necessarily reserved for any certain age. Many people are born with excess facial skin and a lack of facial contour. The characteristic to have jowls — heavy folds of skin in the lower cheek and chin areas — is associated with heredity. Having extra skin on the face gives the appearance of being older than you are, regardless of chronological age. Plus, many young people experience the first noticeable signs of aging as early as their thirties. The rate at which you age is also determined by heredity and changing hormones. In a younger face, a facelift may involve only tightening the skin without working on the deep tissue layers. The results are relative to the elasticity of the skin; the amount of fatty deposits in the face, jowl, and neck areas; the existing jawline definition; and bone structure.

The Two-Layer Facelift

People who read a lot about cosmetic surgery have probably seen recent articles which talk about the "two-layer facelift." These layers refer to the various layers of the face below the skin's surface. The superficial muscles of expression located in the lower part of the face and the muscle in the neck area called the platysma make up one layer. The combination of muscles and fibrous tissue that is just below the fat beneath the skin and neck is referred to as the subcutaneous muscular aponeurotic system (SMAS).

Beneath the SMAS, there is a void space bordered by an inner and outer wall of tissue which is not connected to the bone. As the force of gravity works the inner and outer walls of the SMAS, the facial tissues in the cheeks and around the chin move back and forth and eventually start to sag. This is how facial sagging occurs and how jowls are formed.

The front portion of the platysma muscle controls the cord-like structures which run up and down the neck from the chin to the collarbone. These can be seen when the neck muscles are flexed or strained, and often — with age — flabby, vertical folds develop in the lower face and neck area.

In recent years, plastic surgeons have been particularly concerned with the involvement of the platysma and SMAS in facelift surgery. The facelift of today involves removing or trimming fat from underneath the jaw and the upper neck area, as well as tightening the skin from the lower part of the ears to underneath the chin. But from this point, the surgeon has other options. The platysma muscle can be sculpted by tightening to create a well-defined neck-chin angle. The SMAS, or the muscles and tissues below the fat layer in the skin, can be tightened to reinforce the contour, which may make the facelift longer lasting. These techniques require careful judgment, advanced surgical skill, and a considerable knowledge of anatomy; the platysma and SMAS areas are closely involved with blood vessels, nerves, and the glandular structures which must be protected during the surgery so as not to cause any permanent disruption or damage. The skin is tightened above the muscle and SMAS layers to achieve the overall new contours.

In the past, a facelift was performed by tightening and removing the skin above the layer we call the SMAS. Only the area above the muscles was involved, and the SMAS area was untouched. A few years ago, in an effort to improve the results of facelift, plastic surgeons began incorporating the SMAS into the surgical procedure by pulling it back and anchoring it. The early result in many cases was that the patient's face looked tight and the facelift was conspicuous. This is the origin of some patients' concern that their facelift will look "too pulled or too plastic" and say to their surgeons, "Oh, please don't pull me so tight" or "Please pull as tight as you can." Actually, many patients want to have that "pulled-tight" look, but the best results of facelift are when the face looks very natural and the appearance has not changed. Instead of looking "plastic," the overall effect is that friends and family say, "You look wonderful and very rested. Have you been on vacation?" They know you look terrific, but they can't really tell if you have lost weight, changed your hair, have new makeup, or just look unusually relaxed and happy.

Today, plastic surgeons have become much more experienced manipulating and tightening the SMAS and sculpting the platysma by varying

degrees in order to get very natural-looking results. These advanced facelift procedures help us combine the best of both worlds — a good facelift that is contoured but very natural looking and one that potentially lasts longer than if the deeper layers were not involved at all. Since a facelift is a contouring procedure, enhancement of cheekbones and chin is often recommended.

How Long Does a Facelift Last?

If you have a facelift at fifty-something, which makes you look fortysomething, then when you are sixtysomething, you'll still look younger than if you'd had no facelift at all. Even though a facelift slows down the effects of aging on your appearance, time marches on and we have yet to discover a way to stop the procession.

The lasting results of a facelift vary among individuals — just as the rate at which aging occurs varies among individuals. Some controllable factors help prolong the results, such as avoiding sun exposure, smoking, and excessive alcohol. All the good anti-aging advice written in this book also applies to prolonging the results of a facelift. On the average, people who have repeat facelifts come back for surgery between 5 and 10 years. In some cases, patients who have very heavy, drooping skin around their jaws and in their necks will require a second procedure within a year after the first facelift. This is actually the second stage of the first procedure because the excessive skin sometimes requires extra attention in order to get a good result.

As far as repeat performances go, there is no such thing as too many facelifts. As the patient continues to age, he or she may one day look in the mirror and say, "I'm not as happy as I could be with the way I look." Most patients who have had one facelift are open to doing it again because they know the benefits firsthand.

The results of a facelift are technique dependent. The natural, "good-looking" facelift is the result of properly applied techniques by the experienced, well-trained surgeon.

There are some facial conditions which a facelift cannot correct. The most common are wrinkles, creases, crow's feet, and other fine lines. A facelift can be performed as an adjunct to collagen-replacement therapy, dermabrasion, or chemical peel, which, depending on the nature of the wrinkles, lines, or creases, will offer improvement. A chemical peel or dermabrasion should not be done on skin involved in the facelift itself. (See the sections "Soft-Tissue Augmentation" and "Chemical Peel.")

There is a trend toward performing facelifts at an earlier age today because the better the condition and elastic quality of the skin at the time of surgery, the better the results. Many men and women — especially those in their forties and fifties — are very sensitive to maintaining a youthful appearance because of its positive influence on career. Many more of us do not attach any stigma to cosmetic surgery at any particular age. Since most people are healthier and feel good longer, they naturally want to show it in their looks.

Facelift and Multiple Procedures

As with many other cosmetic surgery procedures, if a patient needs more than one procedure, it may be possible to do multiple procedures at one time.

A facelift alone will not correct bags below or excess skin above the eyes. However, eyelid surgery can be performed at the same time as a facelift to correct the eyelid problem without adding significant extra recovery time or significant additional exposure to anesthesia. Normally, any candidate for a facelift is also a candidate for eyelid surgery because the features of the face usually age and begin to lose elasticity about the same time. (See the section "Eyelid Surgery.")

There are other conditions which a facelift alone will not address. Certain people have inherited characteristics such as a very low forehead and a narrow space between the eyebrows and eyes, or deep furrows between the eyebrows and deep folds of skin in the forehead area which give their faces a tired and angry look. These conditions can be improved with brow-lift surgery, which adds about one hour to the facelift procedure. (See the "Brow-Lift" section.)

In cases where more than one procedure is required and if the surgeon advises that multiple procedures can be performed at one time, many patients prefer to have the surgeries done all at once. Often this approach is more economical in cost and convenience, and many prefer to recoup all at once. One word of warning: Performing simultaneous procedures requires added experience and skill on the part of the plastic surgeon.

Facelift Benefits

The benefits of a properly performed facelift include a younger-looking, more contoured face. The results may turn back the hands of time, but they cannot stop the clock. The aging process continues, even on your face after you have had a facelift. If it helps to put the results into perspective, think of it this way. If you are fifty and have a facelift which makes you look forty, by the time you are sixty, you will still look younger than you would have without any surgery. Patients ask, "If I have a facelift, will I have to keep having them over and over again?" The answer is no, you will not have to have another facelift, although you do have that option. Some people will choose to have several facelifts in the course of a lifetime, especially if they want to maintain very well-defined results.

Facelift Myths

Mini-facelifts which do not require surgery, miracle face-lifting creams, and exercises that produce the same results as a facelift — these are myths that simply have no basis in medical fact, and lead people to waste their money. Nothing replaces facelift surgery, and

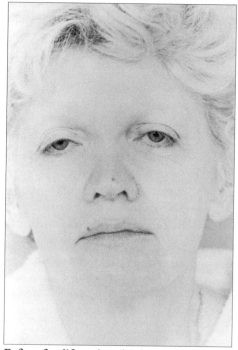

Before facelift and multiple-procedure surgery

nothing accomplishes the same results. Such nonsurgical procedures or products simply do not exist.

Remember, facelift surgery is a very delicate surgical procedure that requires years of experience to learn how to perform. A properly performed facelift requires surgical skill and experience in this specific procedure. The surgery should be performed in a properly equipped operating room under the care of a qualified anesthetist or anesthesiologist and medical staff who are also experienced in supporting this procedure. The recovery and downtime period for facelift surgery is one to three weeks, depending on the patient and

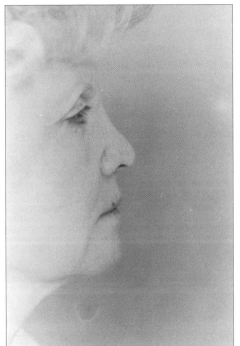

Before facelift and multiple-procedure surgery

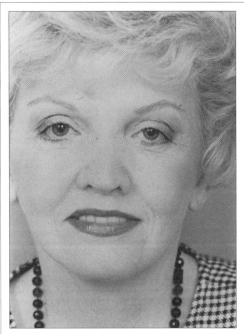

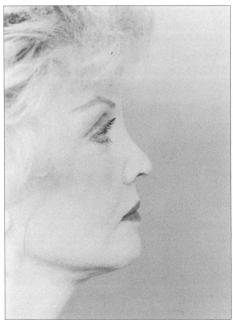

Eleven days after surgery: face and neck lift, brow lift, nose surgery, lower eyelids

extent of the surgery.

The following excerpt is taken from a patient's diary which she kept during the course of her facelift surgery and the recovery period. The diary is followed by her husband's side of the story.

Diary of a Facelift

Stephanie (Age 45)

For starters, I was born with a recessed chin, but I had a lot of excess skin and fat underneath my chin. My mother and my aunt have the very same profile. Looking

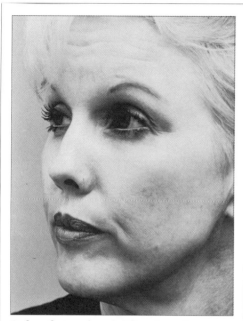

Before face and neck lift and nasal surgery

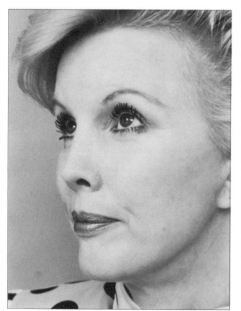

After face and neck lift and nasal surgery

at them and at my own pictures, I realize that this situation becomes more noticeable with age. I look at my high school pictures, wedding pictures, and at recent pictures, and I know it's not my imagination working overtime.

I wasn't sure what could be done because neither my mother nor my aunt has ever done anything to correct the problem. I started checking around, and I asked my dermatologist what he thought. He recommended that I talk to a plastic surgeon, and that's how this all got started. I went to see two different plastic surgeons, and I spent some time examining my options. I knew I wanted to improve my appearance, but I'll admit I was scared. The more I learned, the better I felt, but I was still, well, you could say apprehensive, especially right before the big day, but I went through with it, and I am very glad I did. Here's what happened.

One Week before Surgery

I am scheduled to have a facelift, eyelid and nose surgery, and a chin augmentation. My doctor has shown me a before-and-after image on the computer-imaging system so that I can understand how each procedure is necessary to accomplish the overall result. I have had some lab work, and I have read all the literature. Now, I'm going to try to keep myself busy at home and in the office until the day arrives when I'll actually have the surgery. I'm excited about the final results, but waiting is the worst part for me. Fortunately, Brian is very supportive.

He wants me to do what I want to do, but he keeps telling me that he loves me the way I am. I guess that's why we've stayed married for 22 years.

The Night Before

With all the apprehension and questions I've had in the past few weeks, I am amazingly calm tonight. I'm prepared and ready to get on with the surgery. Tonight I had a nice dinner with my family, and I'm going to bed early. I have to get up at 6:00 a.m. and report to surgery by 7:00. I'm going to sleep, but tonight I'm thinking about the future in a very positive way.

Day 1

On the morning of my surgery, I kept thinking about my children. I was so glad I sent them to Mother's for a few days. They'll be fine. Brian is driving me to the surgicenter, and he's going to wait for me until after the surgery is over.

I was released from the surgicenter about 1:00 p.m., and I couldn't believe that I was awake and aware enough to realize what was happening. I remember absolutely nothing about the surgery itself. The last thing I recall was talking to the nurse, and the next thing I knew I awakened and everything was over.

Brian is taking pictures every day so that I can track my progress. Right now, I have bandages all over my face. I look like a mummy. It's a good thing the kids aren't here. They would make me laugh, and right now I think I'd better just rest.

I know the difference between what I look like today and what I hope to look like in a couple of weeks will be a story in itself.

Day 2

I am swollen and bruised just as they told me I'd be. Surprisingly though, I'm resting pretty comfortably. I can't see to write because the eyelid surgery made my eyes swollen too, but I'm recording my impressions on an audio cassette so I won't forget how I felt each day. Later I'll go back and write everything down in my diary.

Today, the hardest part for me has been lying down and keeping still. I am so accustomed to a busy schedule where I have no time to sit still, so I'm not used to it. Brian is with me because today is Saturday, and he's playing relaxing music, talking to me and even reading me articles out of magazines. I'm going to owe him big time for all this extra special care, but I'll think of something.

Day 3

Today, I feel like watching television, and I can see to read more comfortably. My eyes are still swollen, but they don't hurt. Neither does my nose, which is covered by a small bandage-like splint. It just feels stuffy. I'm not in any pain. I just feel uncomfortable and very tired. I've gotten used to lying still now, and I'm very glad I have this quiet time to rest. My stress level is sure way down, and I'm getting into taking a break. To tell you the truth, the last time I had one was last summer when we went to the beach with the kids, and even that was pretty hectic.

Brian is taking my picture, but I still look swollen and bruised. There hasn't been much change in the way I look, but I definitely am feeling better overall.

Day 6

It's amazing what a difference a few days make. The stitches are out of my eyelids, and the splint is off my nose. I can breathe through my nose comfortably again, and I'm beginning to see some definite improvement in my face. The swelling is going down, and the bruising is starting to lighten up. I'm looking forward to being able to put my contacts back in and being able to drive again. I just didn't realize how independent I really am.

Day 9

Today my doctor sent me to a makeup artist who showed me how to use some special makeup to cover the remaining discoloration under my eyes and on my cheeks. It's unbelievable how much better she made me look and feel. After I went to see her, I met my sister for lunch — yes, lunch in a restaurant. This is the first time I've decided to venture out. I could have gone out a little earlier, but I didn't want to. Now that I know about the makeup, I think I'll feel fine to go just about anywhere.

The most incredible thing happened in the restaurant. My sister and I ran into a friend of ours whom we haven't

seen in at least three months. She kept looking at me, and I became self-conscious because I thought she must have known I'd had surgery. Then all of a sudden she said, "You look really good. Have you lost weight?"

"A few pounds," I replied. My sister — God love her — perked up and said, "Stephanie's been exercising too. She looks great, doesn't she?"

After our friend left the restaurant, my sister and I had a good old-fashioned laugh — the kind we used to have when we were in high school. I'm certainly not going to hide the fact that I've had surgery from my family or real close friends, but I don't want to tell everyone. I just don't want people talking about me. I was absolutely delighted that even now, this woman couldn't tell I'd had anything done.

Day 14 — Morning

I got up early this morning to give myself plenty of time to get ready because I'm going back to work today. I want to look my best because the people at work think I've just been on vacation (except my best friend who knows the whole story). I wonder what they'll say and if they'll notice anything different. Brian and I both think I look great. There is a difference, but I certainly look like myself — I just look a lot better.

Day 14 — Evening

To say that today was interesting is an understatement. Everyone kept asking *me about my vacation and telling me that I looked really good. One woman in my section asked me twice what I'd done differently to my hair. She just couldn't figure it out. When I was leaving and riding down on the elevator, these two women who work on my floor got on the elevator with me and one of them turned and said, "The receptionist says you have a new makeup artist. I'd like to get her name. You look wonderful."*

I laughed to myself and told her I'd give her the name tomorrow. No one said one word about surgery. If they suspected that I'd had anything done, they never said so.

Six Weeks Later

I look in the mirror today, and I am very happy with what I see. My eyes look bright and beautiful, and I love my nose. It just fits my face perfectly. The most exciting change for me is the very subtle change in the overall contour of my face and the definition of my chin. It no longer looks as if my chin and neck run together. There is real definition at my jawline.

I have changed my hair style, and I'm wearing my hair in a way I would never have thought of before. This whole experience has given me more interest in clothes and makeup, too. I feel very experimental with my style these days and much freer to try new ideas. And since everyone thought I had, I went ahead and shed a few pounds.

Brian says he's benefiting from all this too. He's acting like he's got a new

wife. I think he does. I feel terrific, and I'm very energetic about everything. This whole experience has given me a new outlook on life.

While Stephanie was keeping her facelift diary, Brian was busy helping take care of her. He recorded a few thoughts of his own for posterity. Here's what he had to say.

His Side

Brian's Story

Stephanie came home one evening and handed me a computer-printed photo of her profile with a side-by-side view of the same profile with a few changes here and there. She asked me what I thought. Well, I knew she had an appointment with a plastic surgeon to discuss making some changes. I decided I was going to back whatever decision she made, but I was concerned that she get good advice and that she would thoroughly understand what she was getting into.

So when I saw the pictures which represented the changes they wanted to make, I said, "Okay, let's take a hard look at this. First of all, I want you to remember that we've known each other for a very long time, and sure, you've aged a little just like I have. I still find you very attractive, and I love you just the way you are. I understand if you want to improve

161

something, but I don't think it's necessary."

Well, she looked at me with those brown eyes, and I knew that this was something she wanted very much. I sat down with her and we read over the pamphlets the doctor gave her. I told her that I wanted to talk to the doctor too before she made her final decision. Then I looked at her and said, "Okay, let's go for it."

I was with her during the decision-making process, and I helped in the first few days right after surgery. As I write this, it's been three months since the surgery, and I have to say that she does look terrific. She looks younger and prettier. In fact, we knew each other as teenagers, and every time I look at her I can see her back in high school. I think it has to do with the definition in her face and the brightness in her eyes. She's incredibly happy, and that's the most important part. This has made her feel good about herself again. I'll admit she looks years younger to me, but I have to tell you that she really looks better today than she ever has.

Brow-Lift

Brow-lifting is a surgical procedure that involves the forehead and eyebrows. It can be performed as a single procedure, but it is most commonly performed at the same time as a facelift or eyelid surgery to improve a drooping brow, horizontal creases in the forehead,

vertical lines between the eyebrows, and baggy upper eyelids.

The brow-lift is not reserved for the aging face, and not everyone will need this surgical procedure. The conditions which can be improved by a brow-lift are primarily determined by heredity, such as an unusually small space between the eyebrows and the eyes or excess skin that puddles up between the brows at the top of the nose. These inherited features tend to become more pronounced with age, but they rarely — at any age — enhance appearance. As a matter of fact, the vertical folds in the forehead, the closeness of the brows and eyes, and the deep frown lines between the eyes all contribute to a tired- and even angry-looking face, although the person behind the face may not be angry or tired at all.

In this surgical procedure, the skin is incised at or behind the hairline and elevated in order to lift and tighten the forehead area of the face. In the process, the skin and muscle layers are turned down, and the frown muscle is removed so that that muscle will stop pulling on the area above and between the brow which causes the deep lines to form in that area.

Collagen injections are also used in conjunction with brow-lift to fill in and soften the forehead wrinkles and frown lines between the eyebrows. Treatment with injectable collagen improves these lines and creases, but a brow-lift is the necessary solution in most cases where the forehead is low, the eyebrows are drooped, or the brow needs to be lifted.

Chemical peel, and in some cases dermabrasion, also help improve the wrinkles and lines on the forehead and between the eyebrows, but either of these procedures is done at a later time.

Cheek Augmentation, or Malar Augmentation

One of the most distinct aspects of an attractive face is high, prominent cheekbones. You were born either with them or without them, and until recently that's all there was to it. Today, plastic surgery can enhance and enlarge the cheekbones of the face with prosthetic cheekbones molded from a porous plastic substance. Commonly referred to as cheek augmentation, this procedure is used to add definition and contour to a flat facial profile with undefined cheek structure. It can greatly enhance the shape of the face and give the appearance of larger, higher cheekbones. Although cheek augmentation will not tighten facial skin, it can be performed as part of a facelift or as a single procedure.

Chin Augmentation, or Mentoplasty

The size and shape of the chin is also determined by heredity. Sometimes a chin is too small, recedes, or lacks definition. In these cases, a plastic surgeon may recommend a procedure called chin augmentation.

This surgical procedure involves a small, prefabricated prosthetic implant which was developed for surgical

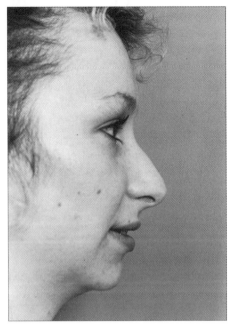

Before nose surgery and chin augmentation

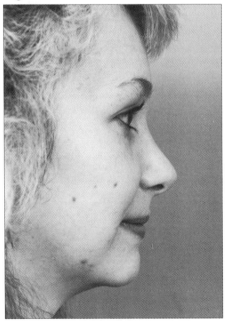

One year after nose surgery and chin augmentation

implantation between the soft tissue and the bone to improve a receding or weak chin by increasing the size and projection of the chin.

A chin augmentation is often done at the same time as a facelift or nasal surgery. (See the sections "The Facelift, or Rhytidetomy" and "Nasal Surgery, or Rhinoplasty.") When the facial contours are enhanced and changed during either of these procedures, it may be necessary to augment the chin and bring it into balance with the other parts of the face.

The chin itself plays an important part in the total facial profile and in the definition of facial contours. If the chin lacks projection and definition, the face does not have a defined profile. As Stephanie described in her facelift diary, "My chin and neck seemed to run together."

Ideally, an attractive facial profile is one in which the forehead, nose, and chin are balanced and in harmony with one another. Most people are not aware of their facial profile as much as they are concerned about a particular feature such as a large nose or protruding ears. However, plastic surgeons are trained to evaluate the three parts of the face and to consider how each part relates to the others. This is what is meant by bringing all facial features into harmony.

There are other surgical procedures involving the chin and the jaw, but traditionally, cosmetic surgeons specialize in aesthetic problems rather than in functional ones.

Eyelid Surgery, or Blepharoplasty

Meet Ed, who at age 48 decided to have eyelid surgery for a very interesting reason.

Ed (Age 47)

One morning I got up and looked in the mirror, and I didn't recognize the person looking back at me. It seemed that all the forty-some-odd years I'd lived caught up with me all at once. The main thing I noticed was my eyes. I had bags underneath my eyes that must have puffed out a half an inch below my eyelashes. I looked like I hadn't slept in months. The wrinkled skin above my eyes hung down so low it was a wonder that I could still see. I figured if I could just fix my eyes, I'd look much better and probably a whole lot younger and healthier. When I looked in the mirror, I saw this tired, old face staring back at me. I'm not a vain person, but I'm going to do something about my eyes, that's all there is to it.

Ed's story is not too unusual, although he did have an excessive amount of extra skin on his upper eyelids which was, in fact, affecting his peripheral vision. Many people of all ages have bags under the eyes and excessive skin which becomes saggy above the eyes. The procedure to correct this problem is the most

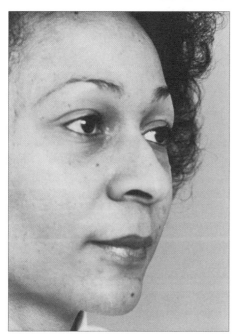

Before upper eyelid and nasal surgery

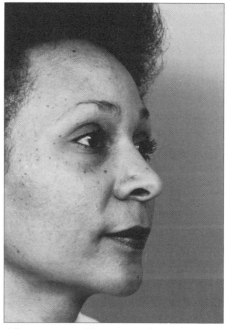

After upper eyelid and nasal surgery

commonly performed facial cosmetic surgery, and it is often the first cosmetic procedure people will have. The majority of eyelid surgeries are performed on people who consider themselves to be in the prime of life and who want their appearance to reflect their youthful outlook. Eyelid surgery is frequently performed at the same time as facelift or surgery to reshape the nose. (See the sections "The Facelift, or Rhytidectomy" and "Nose Surgery, or Rhinoplasty.")

According to 1990 statistics, about 16 percent of the nearly 80,000 cosmetic eyelid surgeries in the United States were performed on men. Of those men, the majority were between the ages of 35 and 64, with average age

being men in their forties. Surgeons and patients alike say that eyelid surgery does more to make a person look younger and fresher than any other type of cosmetic surgery, perhaps because the eyes are such focal points of facial expression. If the eyes look tired, the face looks tired — even when the person behind the eyes is perfectly rested. Before cosmetic surgery, many patients like Ed say the reason they have a hard time accepting how they look in the mirror is because the image they see does not represent how they feel inside.

Cosmetic eyelid surgery is performed on both the upper and lower eyelids, depending on the location and extent of the problem. It is a relatively easy procedure for the patient, and it has a very long-lasting result. Although there is some swelling and bruising in most cases, these conditions disappear within a week or two, and eyelid surgery does not require an extended downtime. The delicate skin around the eyes heals very rapidly, and surprisingly, eyelid skin does not readily scar. If cosmetic eyelid surgery is properly performed, any residual scars are minimal and nicely hidden in the natural creases around the eyes. However, of all cosmetic surgery performed on the face besides nose surgery, eyelid surgery requires the greatest amount of surgical skill and judgment.

What Happens to the Eyes with Age

The thin skin above and below the eyes is often the first part of the face to show evidence of aging. The skin above the eyes expands and gets looser, becoming wrinkled and creased with age. The fatty tissue above and below the eyes tends to increase, even though you may not gain weight or increase your percentage of body fat. The result is sagging "bags" above the eyes and puffy "bags" below the eyes. If the excessive, saggy skin above the eyes hangs down too far, both upward and outward vision can be affected. This condition, also known as "baggy eyelids," tends to be familial, and it is present in people of all ages, even though it becomes more pronounced with age.

A condition called "edema" occurs when extra fluid in the tissues collects in the bags under the eyes. Edema is usually related to water retention associated with hormone changes in women, fluid retention, excessive use of alcohol, smoking, sun exposure, and a lack of sleep. The fluid actually stretches the tissue under the eyes and exaggerates the problem. Surgery will not stop fluid retention, but by reducing the fatty deposit under the eye, the fluid has less space left to collect. Once the fluid and fat are gone, the bags under the eyes disappear to a great extent.

Many people find that the bagginess above and below their eyes becomes a problem as early as their teens or twenties. This is due to genetics rather than aging. At this early age, the bagginess has probably not affected the muscles or stretched the skin. Corrective surgery is normally a very simple operation which removes the fatty tissue in the area and corrects the appearance problem.

Dark Circles under the Eyes

Many people of all ages are concerned with dark circles under their eyes. These dark circles give a tired, sad look, regardless of how a person may really feel. They are caused by shadows and by the dark muscle which shows through from beneath the skin. Blepharoplasty, or eyelid surgery, is not designed to correct the problem of dark circles under the eyes. However, in some cases where excess skin has been removed below the eyes to get rid of the puffy bags, the patient will find that the dark circles are less noticeable.

The following story is told by a

woman who had upper and lower eyelid surgery and whose teenaged daughter also had upper eyelid surgery.

Camille (Age 44) and Laura (Age 17)

I'm not one to worry about a few crow's feet or a wrinkle here and there, but in the last year I really felt like I was looking so much older. I keep myself in very good shape, so my body was actually looking younger than my face, and that bothered me. I went to see a plastic surgeon who told me that I did not need a facelift — certainly not yet, anyway — because I have good contours in my face and good skin tone. What I did need, he said, was eyelid surgery on both my upper and lower lids.

To be frank, I never thought that my eyes were a problem. I guess I just haven't been aware that my eyes were changing. I did notice that when I wore eye shadow and eye liner that it just disappeared because when I opened my eyes, my eyelids were practically nonexistent. I also noticed that when I got bags under my eyes, they didn't go away quickly like they used to. My eyes had a downward turn, and I looked very tired — especially without makeup.

Once the surgeon pointed out what he thought needed to be done, I started to become aware of my upper and lower eyelids. I also noticed that my daughter Laura's upper eyelids were a lot like mine. She told me she never wore eye makeup because it just disappeared. The next time

I went back to the doctor's office, I took her with me.

The result is that we both had our eyelids done, and we both are delighted with the results. Laura needed only to have the hooded skin on her upper lids removed, which opened up her eyes dramatically. She looks so bright eyed and fresh now. She couldn't be happier.

I had the loose skin on my upper lids removed, and the bags under my eyes are completely gone. I am amazed at the overall difference in my face. I look brighter, happy, younger, and so much more rested. This has been good for both Laura and me, and we're having fun with learning how to use eye makeup too.

Both of us had the surgery done over the Christmas holidays, and we were both out and about wearing sunglasses within a week. Neither of us went back to our regular routines for about two weeks, and by that time all the bruising and swelling was gone on both of us.

When I went back to work, everyone commented that I looked great, but no one knew that anything was different. They just kept saying I looked very rested. When Laura went back to school, her friends thought she had changed her makeup technique, and they noticed that she had pulled her hair back out off her forehead in a different style. Even though Laura is an attractive girl, I think this experience has done a lot for her self-confidence. I know it has for mine.

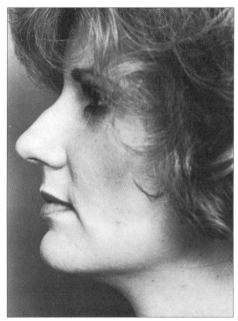
Before nasal surgery to reconstruct the nose

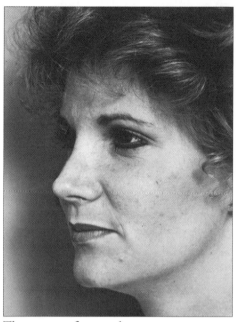
Three years after nasal surgery

Nose Surgery, or Rhinoplasty

The following story tells about a young woman who finally discovered how to correct an appearance problem that had bothered her for a long time.

Bonnie (Age 25)

I know firsthand what people mean when they talk about how you grow up with complexes. It may sound silly, but I had the worst complex about my nose from the time I was about thirteen years old. By the time I was in high school, I was very sensitive about my nose. My dad and I had the same nose. It looked much better

on him than it did on me, that's for sure. No matter how I fixed my hair or what kind of clothes I wore, I was self-conscious about my nose. Every time I saw a picture of myself, I'd say, "If I just didn't have this nose, my face would look much better."

I grew up in a very small town where no one that I had ever heard of knew much about plastic surgery. I know I was isolated, but I didn't realize until I moved to the city to take a job after graduate school that I had the option of having my nose reshaped. I had heard about people having "nose jobs," but for some reason I never related this possibility to me.

A male friend who lived in my

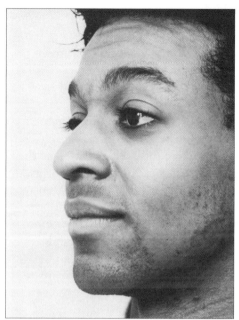

Before nasal surgery to recontour the nose

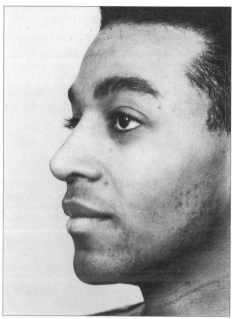

Three months after nasal surgery to recontour the nose

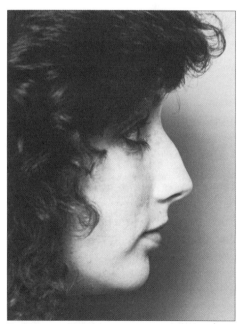

Before nasal surgery to recontour the nose

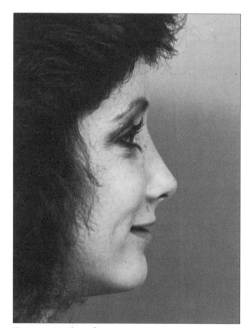

Four months after surgery

apartment building had his nose changed, and that's what got me thinking. I went to see a plastic surgeon shortly thereafter, and the rest is history. I thought the surgery was very painless, and I was out of work a little less than a week. Nothing has ever made such a positive difference in my life. My face looks better, my nose is in proportion to the rest of my face, and my profile from the side is fantastic. This is the best thing I ever did for my self-esteem. I actually like my nose. Will wonders never cease?

Bonnie's story is very similar to those we frequently hear from patients. Besides weight and body size, an unattractive nose is usually the first feature young people are aware of, probably because the nose does most of its growing during the early teenaged years. Parents watch their children go from having child-like noses to having adult-like noses by the time of puberty. The nose has usually reached its mature growth potential by age 15–16, depending on the individual, and nose surgery is not recommended until that growing process is complete.

Very often a pretty girl or a handsome boy will have an unattractive nose which causes an imbalance in the facial harmony. Fortunately, the nose can be reshaped and recontoured to fit the rest of the face. The majority of cosmetic nose surgery is performed through the inside of the nose, even though the results are visible on the outside, except in cases where the nostrils are too large or flared, thus requiring small incisions at the base of the nostril. Nose surgery does not leave any visible scars so long as the corrective work is limited to incisions made inside the nose, which is most commonly the case.

Improving the appearance of the nose consists of many different options. The conditions that make an unattractive nose are as varied as the shapes of noses themselves. For example, a "hump" or "hook" can be removed; an undersized, oversized, wide, plunging, or split tip can be sculpted; nostrils that are too flared can be narrowed; a crooked nose can be straightened; the nose can be made smaller; the bridge of the nose can be built up; the skin and cartilage division between the nostrils (called the columella) can be corrected so that it does not hang down too far; and the angle between the nose and the upper lip can be improved.

Nasal surgery, or rhinoplasty (from the Greek word *rhin*, meaning nose), is the most difficult of all facial cosmetic surgical procedures to perform and the most difficult in which to produce consistently good results. Good results mean the reshaped nose is very natural and in balance with the individual face. Too often noses are made to look too perfect, too chiseled, too sculptured. Even the most attractive natural noses do not look like that. The result of an unnatural-looking nose is that it looks transplanted on the face and is not believable. There are also many unattractive results of nose surgery where the nose looks pinched, too upturned, or too small. The best way to predict a good result is to select a plastic surgeon who is very experienced in this procedure. Ask to see before-and-after photos of the doctor's nose surgery, and try to decide for yourself if the results look natural and balanced.

Many patients feel that reshaping their noses enhances other facial features as well. The reason is that the nose is central to the overall scale and balance of the face. Of course, the nose plays an essential part in the function of the body, affecting breathing, smelling, and vocalizing, but for appearance's sake, the nose is the center of the face, visually bringing together the upper and lower portions of the face. If the size or shape of the nose is out of balance with the other portions of the face, the entire facial structure lacks balance and harmony.

The appearance of the nose is the result of the skin stretched over the cartilage and bony framework. The skin must be draped over this framework. If the skin on the nose is thin, it generally clings to the bone and cartilage beneath it, showing every angle and curve. If the skin is thick, it does not follow the form of the bone and cartilage as readily. Instead, thick skin tends to create a thicker-looking nose that is pudgy and bulbous at the tip. Thinner skin tends to be easier for the surgeon to work with, but improvement is possible for both types.

Surgery of the nose is often functional as well as cosmetic. Many people develop obstructions in the nose that may cause sinus and breathing problems and headaches. It is possible to correct a functional problem and improve the appearance of the nose at the same time.

Ear Surgery, or Otoplasty

Cosmetic surgery to correct large or prominent ears has done much to improve the self-esteem of many men and women of different ages. Children who have big ears or ears that stick out are often ridiculed and as a result grow up feeling terribly self-conscious. This kind of teasing can have a long-lasting effect on self-esteem, and many parents bring their children to a plastic surgeon early in life to correct the problem before emotional scars form.

If the problem of large, protruding ears is left uncorrected, many men and women try to conceal their ears with a hairstyle that covers them. Adult patients who finally decide to correct the problem often say that they are happy with their new look, and that they also experience a feeling of freedom because they no longer feel the need to hide or cover up their ears.

Ears protrude when the elastic cartilage that folds the ear toward the head is either poorly developed or improperly formed. In this procedure, the ears are positioned closer to the head by reshaping the cartilage or supporting tissue. There are small incisions placed behind the ears so that any remaining scars will be concealed in a natural skin crease.

In most cases, large or protruding ears are obvious at a very young age.

Fortunately, cosmetic ear surgery can be performed by about age five or six, when at least 80 percent of the growth of the ear has occurred, and surgery will not interfere with any future ear growth. When the ears are corrected prior to a child entering school, the surgery helps eliminate potential psychological trauma.

No two ears are alike, so in the course of the surgery, each ear must be treated on an individual basis. After surgery, no two ears look exactly alike either, but the surgeon will attempt to balance them as closely as possible. Some cosmetic problems involving ears affect only one side of the head, or the problem is different on each side.

Although the majority of cosmetic ear surgery is performed on children, it can be performed on patients of all ages. There are other cosmetic problems which primarily bother adults. The earlobe can be too long or it can become stretched with age or by wearing heavy pierced earrings. Sometimes the earlobes become wrinkled and creased with age, and for people who have had cosmetic surgery of the face, such as a facelift or chemical peel, and who otherwise look young for their age, the wrinkled earlobes can be very unattractive. Surgery can reduce the size of the earlobe and tighten the stretched earlobe. A peel or dermabrasion can improve the wrinkled-looking earlobe in order to help match the quality of the earlobe skin to the rest of the face.

Most cosmetic ear surgery is performed under local anesthesia on an out-patient basis, except in cases of small children. The patient is usually awake, but cannot feel the surgery once the anesthesia has taken effect. However, in most cases with teenagers or adults, mild sedation is used. Most children deal very well with the surgery because they are already aware that their ears are unattractive, and they want to have the problem corrected as much as their parents do.

Cosmetic Surgery for the Body

Male and female bodies have obvious gender differences which are a part of the natural evolution of the sexes. The male body is typically characterized by bigger bones and more muscle mass, with proportionately longer legs and feet, broader shoulders, longer arms, bigger chests, stronger skulls, and thicker and sturdier jaws.

Women, on the other hand, are born with more fat cells than men. Women have a wider pelvis, a more slender waist, thicker thighs, a longer belly, a narrower chest, protruding breasts and buttocks, shorter legs, narrower shoulders, fleshier lips, and less body hair.

While these are only some of the typical gender differences, they form the basis of many of the physical differences in the forms and figures of each sex. They also form the basis for many traditional body image concepts upon which we place a great deal of value.

It is human nature to compare ourselves to one other and especially to other members of our own sex. Culture and society have always influenced our ideas of attractive male and female body types, even though there is an increasing acceptability of individual differences and personal preferences. But no matter what kind of body you have or want to have, and regardless of what kind of body you are attracted to in a mate, the physical appearance and condition of our bodies play a key role in self-esteem and physical health.

Your body makes an impression on others just as your face does, and your body language is a big part of your communications package. From the psychological perspective, the key role the body seems to play is in the arena of self-acceptance. Those who feel good about their bodies have a higher level of self-acceptance and a greater sense of freedom of expression. That is why exercise and fitness are so important. Most of us do not, by any means, have perfect bodies, but when we are fit and are taking good care of ourselves, our self-esteem seems to soar.

Some inherited body features and acquired conditions cannot be improved with exercise or proper nutrition, and these are the problems that cosmetic surgery was developed to help. There are also some body features and conditions that — with age — need a little help in order to keep them looking as good and feeling as young as possible.

The next several sections provide a general overview of cosmetic surgery procedures which offer improvement for body contours and body proportions. It is important for the various features and portions of the body to be in balance and harmony with each other, and very often bringing all parts of the body into scale makes the positive difference. As with cosmetic surgery of the face, keep in mind that cosmetic surgery can do wonderful things for the figure or the physique, but the results are only as good as the skill of the surgeon performing the procedure.

The following story comes from a patient whose figure and frame of mind were enhanced by liposuction. For years she tried every exercise and work-out routine, but there were certain spot problems which simply would not go away.

Marilyn (Age 33)

I inherited the bottom-heavy figure that all the women on my mother's side of the family have. I am very small on the top and pear-shaped on the bottom, so in order to get the lower half of my body in proportion with the upper part of my body, I have to be so thin that my face looks like a skeleton — and even then I can't get rid of the saddlebag thighs. In a tight-fitting pair of jeans, I look like I am wearing jodhpurs. I don't ride horses, and I absolutely hate my thighs. When I heard that maybe there was hope from lipo-suction, I was thrilled because I have done every kind of exercise regularly, including jogging and weight lifting, to no avail.

I found a good doctor and checked both his references from other patients and his experience with liposuction. I set up the appointment and couldn't wait. I decided to have liposuction on my outer and inner thighs and the lower portion of my buttocks.

After the fact, I was very black and blue for about four days, and I was pretty sore in the areas where the fat had been suctioned, but soon the discoloration began to fade and the soreness began to go away. Altogether, I only missed three days of work because I had the liposuction done on a Friday, which gave me the weekend days to get over the main soreness and feeling of being tired.

I'm very happy with the result. It's been six months, and I have not put the fat back on in those areas. I did not lose weight, but I definitely lost inches in my thighs, which is exactly what I wanted. I look much better in jeans and straight skirts, and I feel better all over.

Liposuction: Lipolysis or Lipectomy (Also Known as Body Contouring)

Marilyn's story is a good example of why liposuction has become such a popular surgery. It is not a substitute for weight loss or exercise. It offers improvement for those who exercise and watch their weight but who cannot get rid of extra fat in problem areas.

Liposuction was first developed in France in the mid-1970s.

In the last several years, liposuction has become the most in-demand cosmetic surgery procedure in this country. According to recent statistics from the American Society of Plastic and Reconstructive Surgeons, 109,080 liposuction procedures were performed in the United States in 1990, a 95 percent increase over the 1981 total.

The various names for this elective procedure are generally synonymous. Body contouring is the first advancement to come along that offers assistance in changing the contours of the body without making large surgical incisions. However, such medical progress does not mean that fat suctioning is easy to perform. Successful results depend on a surgeon's keen understanding of anatomy and physiology, surgical judgment, and successful experience in performing previous liposuction procedures.

Many doctors who do not have surgical training perform liposuction, and many health-threatening complications have occurred when these doctors lacked the knowledge and experience to handle problems which arose. Considerable media coverage of problems surrounding liposuction has raised public awareness of the importance of selecting an experienced surgeon to perform the procedure.

In cosmetic procedures, liposuction is used to remove excess fatty deposits from various areas of the body and stubborn pockets of fat which collect in specific areas. It is used to balance one part of the body with another and to bring all portions of the body into

Before liposuction

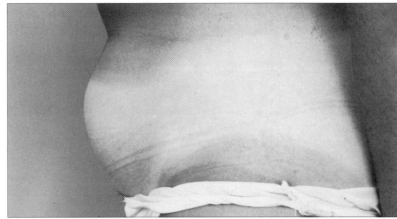

After liposuction

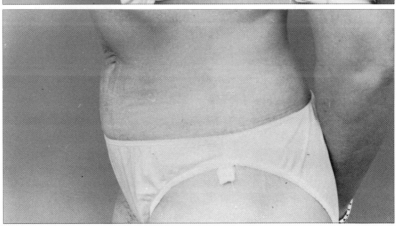

harmony with each other. Body contouring is typically performed on patients of relatively normal weight and body build to reduce disproportionately large hips and thighs (saddlebags, which are common in women) or a protruding abdomen (pot belly), or to remove excess fat around the waist (love handles) or from the buttocks. It is also used to remove fat on the arms, calves, and knees, and neck and above the breasts, from the jowls, and under the chin.

Fat-suctioning techniques are also basic to other types of surgery. They are used to remove fatty tumors, as a combination procedure in face- and neck-lift surgery, and to remove fat from underneath a double chin. It is also used in breast-reduction surgery to get rid of excess fat underneath the arms.

The best results from liposuction occur in areas where there is reasonable muscle tone, where skin has good elastic quality, and where intra-abdominal fat is not excessive. In cases where there is a significant loss of tone and elasticity, a good result requires a combination of both liposuction and surgery; in order to get an attractive body contour, the patient needs both fat suctioning to remove the fatty deposits and a surgical tightening to remove the excessive, loose skin.

Liposuction is performed by inserting a very small instrument called a cannula, a narrow tube with holes near its end, underneath the skin into the channel of fat. The surgeon passes the cannula back and forth in a smooth, steady, motion, and the fat is literally suctioned away through a strong suction machine that is attached to the cannula. Since the cannula is quite small, the incisions in the skin are also small and usually heal very quickly with minimal scarring. There are normally two to three incisions made in each area of the body where fat is to be suctioned. The procedure is usually performed under local anesthesia with sedation, on an out-patient basis, and takes about 45 minutes to 2 hours, depending on the extent of suctioning to be done.

In the process of suctioning away fat, the fatty deposits are broken up and vacuumed away. In removing fat from the body, we are actually removing fat cells too. The logical question that always comes up is, "How do fat cells affect body weight?"

When you gain weight, the number of cells containing fat increases. We believe that the fat-suctioning procedure actually removes fat cells and that they will not return to any great extent. There have been some basic studies to support this theory, but it has not been solidly proven as of yet. Many patients say that they did not gain the weight back in the area that was suctioned and that having the procedure was a positive motivator for increasing exercise and following a smart eating plan.

Cellulite

Cellulite is predominately a problem for women, who, unlike men, package fat in a way that causes a visible rippling effect in the skin. Cellulite collects primarily on hips and buttocks. It is best described as small compartments attached to the under surface of the skin which are overstuffed with fat cells. Imagine that a collection of fat cells is like a room where fat is stored. When the room is too full, the walls bulge past their capacity. The rippling effect of cellulite on the skin is caused by too many fat cells overfilling the fibrous compartments. In essence, cellulite is like any other fat, but its appearance is different because of the way it is stored.

There are some unhealthy habits which contribute to the cellulite collection — such as lack of exercise, too much alcohol, eating chocolate and fried foods, and smoking cigarettes — but this condition basically affects women who have inherited the tendency to have cellulite. It also has to do with the different ways in which women and men store fat and the ways in which skin is attached.

The skin in women attaches to underlying muscle by thin parallel cords. These cords are not very flexible, and the fat that women gain spills over into the ridges between the cords. The result is a textured surface of fat on the skin which is very hard to get rid of, no matter what you do. Most men store fat differently from women. Their connective tissue is a very tightly woven layer of strands. Men store fat in a smooth layer, and there are no ridges into which the fat can spill over. In women's bodies, the connective tissue which clings to the fat and holds it in place contributes to the "cellulite spill" and allows it to create bulges and fatty deposits.

Diet is a major factor in the cure of cellulite. When weight is lost, the pressure on the walls of the compartments where fat is stored lessens. A low-fat diet that is high in complex carbohydrates and moderate in protein content is the best answer to cellulite control. Low-fat diets lower estrogen production. Estrogen, the female hormone, promotes fat buildup and increases hunger and water retention.

Liposuction can help because reducing the amount of fat volume helps to reduce the pressure on bulging fat, but liposuction is not a cure-all. Liposuction is basically a contouring procedure which is designed to get rid of those last bulges that dieting will not reduce, but it does not attack the cellulite directly.

Tummy Tuck, or Abdominoplasty

Many of us inherit the tendency to store fat in the stomach, just as others store fat in the thighs, buttocks, upper arms, or midriff area. Where you store excess fat is largely determined by genetics, and your individual fat patterns determine your body type. (See "Which Body Type Are You?")

For those who want to improve the appearance of the abdominal area, the surgical procedure commonly known as tummy tuck may be right for you. The abdominal problem generally falls into two categories: a stretching of the abdominal skin caused by recurrent weight gain and loss and a stretching of the abdominal muscles with one or more pregnancies.

Abdominoplasty is not a procedure to be taken lightly because it is considered major surgery and is more extensive and involved than other cosmetic surgeries. It includes separating the skin from the muscle wall, tightening the muscle of the abdominal wall, fat suctioning — if necessary in adjacent areas — and surgical excision or removal of excess skin. A tummy tuck also involves making a hip-to-hip incision and sometimes a vertical incision. Although the horizontal one can be located below the waistline across the top of the pubic hair, it will leave a noticeable scar even after healing has occurred. The scars will eventually fade and improve but are nonetheless associated with this surgery.

The recovery time from this surgery is also longer than with other cosmetic procedures. Depending on the patient and the individual rate of recovery, a tummy tuck patient should allow about three to four weeks away from work and normal social activity.

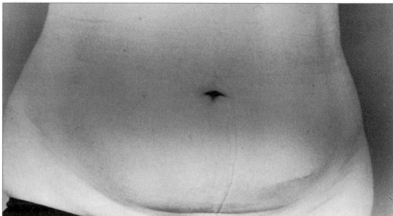

Before abdominoplasty

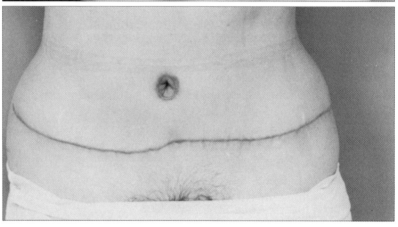

After abdominoplasty

In spite of these considerations, many patients who are concerned about the appearance of their tummies, in or out of clothes, say that to have a flatter, firmer stomach once again (or for the first time ever) is worth the surgery. A tummy tuck can accomplish results that diet, exercise, and liposuction cannot.

The Female Breast

There is no other female body part that commands so much attention or has greater influence on a woman's sense of self than the breast. Let's take a good look at these miraculous creations of both form and function.

The breast is actually a gland which contains fatty tissue, milk ducts, lobes or clusters of tiny sacs, and a network of lymph vessels. The breast contains no muscles, which explains why women cannot increase the size of the breast by bulking the muscles (pectorals) behind the breasts.

The breast nipple contains sensory nerve endings. Sexual stimulation causes the nipple to harden, the pigmented

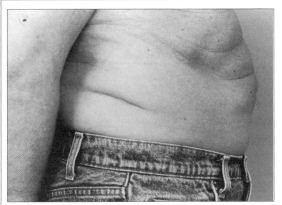
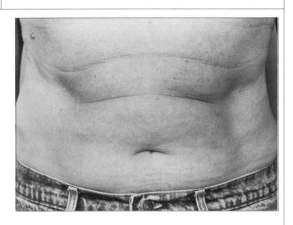

Before abdominal surgery

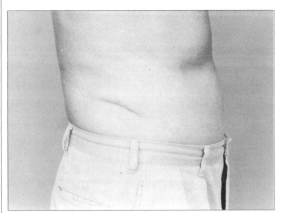
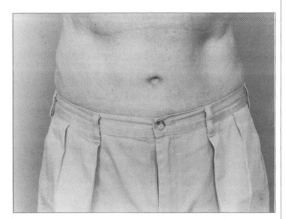

Seven months after surgery

area around the nipple (called the areola) to enlarge, and the breast to swell.

Like the rest of the body, the breasts change during different stages of life and with age. During pregnancy, for example, the milk glands which are located just behind the nipple respond to two pituitary hormones and begin to produce milk within the lobes, or clusters of tiny sacs. The hormones which spark all this activity are prolactin, which stimulates the milk production within the glands, and oxytocin, which

stimulates the milk to move through the milk ducts to the nipple and into the baby's mouth.

Nursing a baby can be a healthy, wonderful experience for both mother and child, and many experts think that the nursing process even offers some protection for the mother from breast cancer later in life. However, as the breast gland expands and becomes engorged with milk, the breasts become enlarged, and the skin stretches to accommodate the larger gland and the supply of milk. This expansion process can cause the appearance of the breast to change.

After the mother weans the nursing baby, the breast gland involutes (goes back to its pre-pregnancy state) and sometimes becomes even smaller. The skin which has stretched to accommodate the engorged breast rarely reverts to its original elastic condition. This is what causes the breast to sag after a mother has nursed a child. With each pregnancy and lactation (when the breast produces milk), the breasts become engorged, the skin stretches, and the gland involutes. Each time this cycle occurs, additional pressure is put on the skin covering the breasts, and like all skin that is stretched and restretched, the skin over the breasts becomes more inelastic with repeated stressful action. The result is breasts that are less firm and erect than before childbearing and nursing.

Another change occurs throughout the productive years before menopause. The breasts may secrete fluid that occasionally leaks from the nipple. More than 90 percent of all nipple discharges are normal, but because nipple discharge can be an early warning sign of cancer, many women become unnecessarily alarmed. Of course, it is always advisable to check with your doctor regarding this or any other suspicious breast condition — especially if the nipple is sore, looks abnormal, or is tender to the touch.

In the years before menopause, there are regular cyclical changes which occur in breasts as the body responds to the changing levels of the hormones known as estrogen and progesterone.

These hormones may cause premenstrual lumps to appear in the breasts and then to disappear within a few days of menstruation. As menopause approaches, cysts and irregular densities sometimes appear and premenstrual breast tenderness may increase.

Later during menopause, decreasing levels of estrogen and progesterone cause breast tissue to shrink. Firm tissue is replaced by fatty tissue, and the breasts become softer. The skin becomes stretched in relation to the degree of change that has occurred in the breasts over the years.

As women get older they are at increasing risk of developing breast cancer, and by far the greatest number of breast cancers originate in the mammary ducts which carry milk to the nipple. Most breast cancers are discovered by mammogram or by touch — even though a tumor does not show up on a mammogram for one to five years or by touch for one to seven years.

Fortunately, women today are aware — more than ever — of the importance of having mammograms and conducting self-exams. The most important part of breast disease is facing the facts and taking control over both the prevention and detection processes as well as the treatment process should breast disease occur.

Breast cancer is on the rise in this country, and the statistics have increased to indicate that one in nine women will have breast cancer in her lifetime. As discouraging as these rising figures are, there is good news too.

The improved rate of early

detection of breast cancer and advanced treatment techniques and procedures have dramatically improved the survival rates of breast-cancer patients. By detecting breast tumors early and using improved treatment methods, the number of mastectomies (surgical procedure to remove the breast) are also decreasing. According to figures from the Dana Farber Cancer Institute in Boston, among women under 50 years old with breast cancer, 78.7 percent live at least five years and 66.2 percent live ten years. For women older than 50, the numbers are similar: a five-year survival rate of 78.6 percent and a ten-year survival rate of 61.7 percent. Longer-term predictions have not yet been made.

The women who are most at risk statistically are those who are over 40, have a family history of the disease, never had children or had children after age 30, began having periods before age 12, went through menopause after age 55, or belong to low-income groups where mammography is not readily available.

Funding for mammography is a hot issue today because in many states insurance companies and third-party insurers are not required by law to provide coverage of screening mammography. As a result, many women — particularly low-income women — are not screened early enough. A 1990 report, "Poverty and Breast Cancer in New York City," discovered that 60 percent of breast-cancer cases in women of low incomes, which were diagnosed in 21 hospitals around the city, were detected in advanced or late stages.

Early detection and treatment of breast cancer is crucial for all women. Women are advised to become very familiar with their breasts and to become accustomed to changes which tend to occur on a monthly basis so that they can better detect any unusual change. If an unusual mass is discovered in the breast, it is vitally important to consult with a surgeon who specializes in breast disease without delay. It is a good plan to see a specialist who routinely diagnoses and treats breast cancer. Your gynecologist, internist, or plastic surgeon will be able to refer you.

The surgeon will order a mammogram of both breasts and possibly a sonogram, which is a painless imaging procedure that uses sound waves to distinguish fluids from solids. If there is a cyst or fluid-filled lump in the breast, the surgeon will draw out the fluid with a very fine needle, which reduces the swelling caused by the lump. Less than 1 percent of these types of cysts or lumps are cancerous, but the doctor may still order a test on the liquid removed from the breast.

If the lump in the breast is solid, the lump will be surgically removed from the breast (biopsy), and a pathology examination will be per-formed to determine the status of the lump. About 80 percent of all lumps which are biopsied prove to be benign or harmless, but careful diagnosis is absolutely necessary in order to insure successful detection and treatment of possible breast disease.

In cases where the biopsy is positive, which means breast cancer has been found, the patient should begin immediately to work with a team of medical specialists, including a pathologist, one or more oncologists, a general surgeon, a radiation therapist, and a plastic surgeon who specializes in the breast.

Anyone who is concerned about breast disease or who has a breast problem should call a local chapter of the American Cancer Society for referrals to both doctors and support groups who can help and provide valuable sources of educational information.

Cosmetic Breast Surgery

There are various types of cosmetic breast surgery that can accomplish different objectives. Although many people disapprove of or have no interest in cosmetic surgery on the breasts, many women who have small breasts, have very large breasts, or have lost one or both breasts to cancer say that these procedures are very positive factors in their lives. Some men who have excess fatty tissue in the breast or chest area also claim their lives and their physiques have been enhanced by modern cosmetic surgical procedures.

Breast Augmentation, or Augmentation Mammaplasty

The cosmetic procedure known as breast augmentation is used to enlarge and enhance small or underdeveloped breasts, to balance asymmetry (unequal size or shape) of the breasts, or to improve saggy breasts which have atrophied after childbearing.

There are several possible surgical approaches to breast augmentation, most of which are performed under local anesthesia on an out-patient basis. The most common approaches involve a surgical incision which is made in one of two places: in the natural crease of the breast just above where it touches the chest or around the lower border of the areola, the dark skin that surrounds the nipple. In some cases, the incision can be made in the armpit. The decision of where to make the surgical incision depends on the surgical technique involved, the patient's anatomy and preference, and the plastic surgeon's judgment.

Having made the incision, the surgeon lifts the breast tissue up to create a pocket either directly under the breast gland or underneath the pectoral muscle, depending again on the surgical technique selected.

Once the pocket is made, the surgeon places a breast implant or prothesis into the pocket and closes the incision with a few sutures. The breast implant is a breast-shaped bag of clear silicone rubber filled with either a saline (salt water) solution, a silicone gel, or both. After surgery, which normally takes about one to two hours, a gauze dressing may be applied over the breasts or the patient may be placed in a surgical bra. The surgical incisions cause scars, but the surgeon will attempt to conceal the incisions in natural skin creases so that once they heal, they will

Before breast augmentation

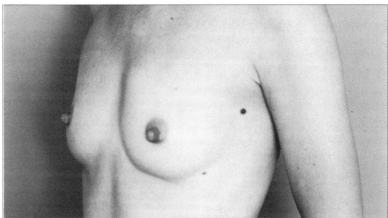

Two years after breast augmentation

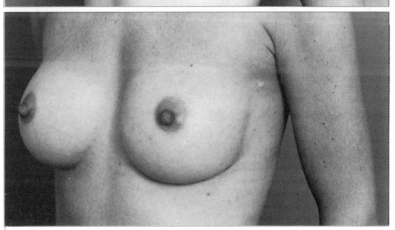

be less obvious. At first, scars appear very red, but in time, discoloration fades and scars become much less noticeable.

The most common problem associated with breast implants is called capsular contracture, which is an annoying condition that occurs when the implanted prosthesis becomes firm caused by scar contracture which occurs around it. The breast becomes hard because the body forms a fibrous capsule which contracts around the implant. Treatment involves breast massage, breast compression to break the capsule, and in some cases, a second surgical procedure to cut the scar tissue surgically and in some cases replace the existing implant with a new or different type.

Recent government investigations and media coverage have brought attention to the issue of the safety of silicone gel used in breast implants. Manufacturers of the implant devices have produced extensive studies involving breast implants which have been used in over two million women. Dow Corning Wright, which first developed the silicone substance, has documented over 700 studies involving breast implants which have been used for over thirty years. To date, all indications are that silicone is safe, but the FDA has required manufacturers to conduct further studies and to produce further findings which support long-term safe results. As this book goes to press, the FDA's final ruling on silicone gel breast implants has not been decided. Contact your doctor for the most up-to-date information.

The substance silicone is used in many devices and products other than breast implants. It is used to insulate cardiac pacemakers, to coat hypodermic needles, and in routine, over-the-counter medications such as laxatives. Silicone is also used in other implant devices such as artificial finger joints and testicular implants. According to studies conducted on various types of implants, there is no evidence that the body produces antibodies to silicone when it is present.

There are three basic types of breast implants which have been used to date, all of which are constructed of clear silicone rubber. One type has a single chamber filled with silicone gel, another has a single chamber filled with a saline solution, and a third type has a double chamber — one inside the other — with silicone gel in the inner chamber and saline solution in the outer chamber.

A national survey of women who have had breast augmentation for cosmetic or reconstructive reasons was recently conducted by Market Facts, Inc., of Chicago. The survey selected a panel of 100,000 households to repre-

sent the nation's consumer population and screened them for the presence of women who had breast implants. Detailed questionnaires were completed by 592 women, of which 65 percent had breast implants for cosmetic reasons and 35 percent had breast implants for reconstruction after cancer or other disease. Overall, these implants had been in place for an average of eight years at the time of the survey.

The survey's results showed that an overwhelming majority are satisfied with the results of their breast implants and would choose to have the surgery again. As a matter of fact, 92.5 percent of the respondents said they were satisfied with their results, and 82 percent said that without a doubt they would have the surgery again.

The survey also revealed the three most common reasons these women elected to have breast implants for cosmetic reasons:

• 93 percent desired a more proportionate figure

• 83 percent desired a more appealing appearance

• 76 percent desired to boost their self-confidence

Women who had breast implants as reconstruction after breast cancer surgery also listed their primary reasons for choosing to have breast implants:

• 90 percent desired to be free from the need to wear an external prosthesis

- 79 percent wanted to have breast implants so as not to be constantly reminded about their breast cancer

- 75 percent wanted to feel whole again

Breast Lift, or Mastopexy

A breast lift is typically performed to correct sagging or loose breasts or breasts that have lost volume and elasticity after childbirth and nursing. This cosmetic surgical procedure can also reduce the size of the areola, the dark pink skin surrounding the nipple. It is commonly performed under local or general anesthesia, depending on the size of the breasts and the changes to be made, on an out-patient basis.

In this operation, the surgeon makes incisions following the natural contour across the breast and around the areola. These incisions define the area of skin to be removed and the new, higher location of the nipple. Next, skin formerly located on the sides of the breast is brought around and pulled together to reshape the breast. Sutures close the incisions and restore the breast contour. In cases where there is minimal sagging of the breasts, a modified procedure can be used to surgically remove only skin from the large areola and its immediate surrounding area. For women desiring larger breasts, breast augmentation can be performed at the same time as a breast-lift procedure.

Although there are scars from the surgical incisions, they usually fade with time and become less visible. Any scarring would not be visible in low-cut clothing, a bathing suit, or a bra. The results of a breast lift are firmer breasts which do not sag as they did before and a more youthful body appearance.

Brenda (Age 40)

I have had three children, and I wouldn't trade them for anything, but I often tease that I traded my body for each of them. I have always been big busted, but with each pregnancy and each passing year, my breasts got even larger.

My oldest child is ten, and my youngest is six. They're all in school this year, and I have a newfound freedom that has made this an interesting year for me.

I made a decision to have a breast reduction. At first, my husband fought it, but eventually he came around to understand how I felt. I was so tired of carrying around such big breasts, and they really gave me problems — such as severe back and shoulder pain that got so bad that sometimes I just wanted to stay in bed, which is not like me at all.

My clothes never fit right, and I hated wearing bathing suits or tee shirts. I was tired of having to be limited to two-piece outfits because nothing in a one-piece outfit that fit the top ever fit the bottom. I always had to buy one-size top and one-size bottom. I couldn't find dresses, and clothes generally made me feel self-conscious about my figure. There was no way to disguise my so-called full figure.

So, I made the decision to have a breast reduction, and I cannot remember ever being so happy with any decision I

185

have ever made. It took a couple of weeks out of my regular routine, and for the first week, I was sore and uncomfortable. After I felt better, the first thing I did was to go out and buy a new outfit and some new lingerie. I thought about having a bra-burning party, but the new, smaller-size bras I bought are so beautiful that I just tossed out the old harnesses instead. My husband has really come around, and he admits that he likes the way I look now because he says I look very trim and much more shapely.

Breast Reduction: Reduction Mammaplasty

Brenda's story expresses a view shared by many breast-reduction patients. They describe themselves as "uncomfortable," "self-conscious," and "never having clothes to wear that fit comfortably." Large, heavy breasts put a strain on shoulders and backs and cause many women to have grooves on their shoulders where bra straps have cut into the skin. Many women have poor posture as a result of carrying the excess weight of large breasts.

The size and shape of breasts are as individual as women themselves. Breast size is hereditary, and weight gain can increase the fatty tissue around the breasts. A few women wish for larger breasts, and a few want firmer breasts, but a large number of women who have large, heavy breasts definitely want smaller breasts. In fact, breast-reduction patients are among the most satisfied patients of all those who have any cosmetic surgery procedure.

The most common breast-reduction surgery involves an incision made around the areola or the dark-skin area around the nipple. Another incision descends from the nipple to the fold of skin underneath the breast. A third incision is located under the breast. It is placed in the fold of the skin which runs between the lower breast and the chest wall. These incisions join together to form a pattern that is in the shape of an anchor. In the case of very long, thin breasts or unusually large breasts, it is sometimes desirable to remove the nipples and replace them as skin grafts onto the newly reduced breast mound so that the nipples will be positioned properly and in balance with the new breast size.

Breast-reduction surgery normally takes about two hours. It is performed under general anesthesia and can be performed on an out-patient basis. After surgery, the breasts are supported in gauze dressing or a special bra which is worn for about two weeks. Most patients can return to work after about a week but must limit physical activities for a longer period, depending on the extent of the surgery. There is some extended care required in cases involving nipple grafts.

Breast reduction and nipple grafting usually result in some degree of numbness around the nipple. There are scars which result from the incisions made. These scars are very noticeable at first but usually fade and blend with the rest of the skin in time. Unfortunately, some degree of the scarring is permanent.

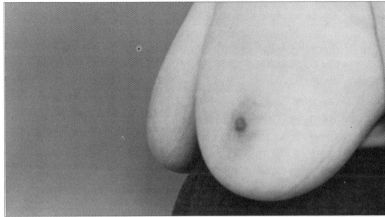

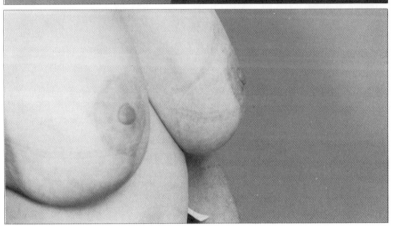

Male Breast-Gland Reduction, or Gynecomastectomy

Many men recognize the problem, but many say they did not know there was a way to solve it. That's why one of the most increasingly popular cosmetic surgery procedures for men is gynecomastectomy, which involves removal of the breast gland and excess fatty tissue in the breast and chest area where men tend to deposit fat.

Some men are born with large breast glands or excessive amounts of fat in this area, and many men who gain weight store fat in this area. As men age, the tendency to store fat in the breast area increases. Also, many men have developed excess muscle tissue in this area as a result of weight training. As they age or discontinue the weight training, the muscle can be replaced by fat.

Male patients who have this chest-contouring surgery are highly satisfied because men feel that an enlarged breast

187

area does not match the masculine image they have of themselves. Many men who have this surgery are delighted with the improved results; they claim that it helped increase self-esteem because it improved their appearance both in and out of clothes.

The surgery involves a semi-circle incision which is made around the dark pigmented area of the nipple. An incision in this area usually heals very nicely, and the shading produced by the change in pigmentation between the nipple and the flesh-colored skin helps to conceal any remaining scar. Once the incision has been made, the breast gland is surgically removed and the excess fat is tapered and recontoured. The incision is then closed with a few sutures. In older patients and in patients where the breast gland is not too large and is predominantly fat, liposuction can be used instead of surgery to remove the gland and fatty tissue.

In most cases, this procedure is performed on an out-patient basis, and local or general anesthesia can be used. The patient can return to work and normal social activity within five to seven days with limited upper-arm and lifting activities for two to four weeks.

EPILOGUE
Maximizing
Potential

The best reward any doctor can ever have comes from helping others feel better. In our practices, we have the great fortune of helping people feel good about themselves. To watch someone grow and develop his or her potential right before your very eyes is very inspiring —like watching a flower bloom through time-lapse photography.

Potential is something each of us has. We are born with it, and as we live our lives, we continue to develop it. It is as simple as learning to take advantage of information and as challenging as reaching for ambitious goals. All in all, developing potential is something we owe ourselves.

There is a great correlation between health and potential because they are the components involved in creating the "quality" of our lives. Protecting and promoting health and understanding and

developing personal potential are the major determining factors involved in making the most of ourselves and of our lives.

The purpose of this book is to encourage everyone who reads it to be the best he or she can be. This is a great challenge in life and a very valuable experience. It is possible to make use of human potential and to expand yourself into a fuller circle of happiness, health, and contentment.

REFERENCES

BOOKS

Brenton, Myron. *Aging Slowly.* Pennsylvania: Rodale Press, Emmaus, 1983.

Evans, William, Ph.D., and Irwin H. Rosenburg, M.D. *Biomarkers: The 10 Determinants of Aging You Can Control.* New York: Simon & Schuster, 1991.

Hauser, Gayelord. *New Treasury of Secrets: Your Passport to a Better Way of Living.* Toronto: Doubleday Canada Ltd., 1991.

Madry, Bobbi Ray. *Standard Textbook for Professional Estheticians.* 5th ed. Israel Rubinstein, Milady Publishing Corporation, 1986.

Morris, Desmond. *Manwatching: A Field Guide to Human Behavior.* New York: Harry N. Abrams, Inc., 1977.

Passwater, Richard A., Ph.D. *The New Super Nutrition.* New York: Pocket Books, 1991.

PERIODICALS

"Ageless Beauty." *McCall's.* vol. 119, no. 1 (October 1991): 118–19.

"Anti-Aging News." *Longevity.* vol. 1, no. 6 (March 1989): 8.

Blakeslee, Sandra. "The True Story Behind Breast Implants." *Glamour* (August 1991): 186–89, 230–31.

Britton, A. G. "Know Thyself." *Self* (November 1991): 125–33, 186.

Byrd, Beverly. "Your Skin and the Sun." *Dermascope* (March/April 1989): 34.

Costigan, Kelly. "Up to Your Ears in Ears?" *In Health.* vol. 5, no. 3 (May/June 1991): 26, 28.

Crichton, Michael. "Happiness Is . . ." *Self* (August 1991): 88.

Davis, Lisa. "Breast Implants: Two Million Guinea Pigs?" *In Health.* vol. 5, no. 5 (September/October 1991): 32–34.

Drexler, Madeline. "The Breast." *Lear's* (August 1991): 49-55, 94.

Eller, Daryn, and Margaret Pierpont. "Keeping Your Body Younger Longer." *Longevity* (October 1991): 58, 60, 62, 64.

Ferrara, Dan. "Working Hard or Hardly Working?" *In Health.* vol. 5, no. 3 (May/June 1991): 96.

Freeburg, Maureen. "Can Money Buy Happiness?" *Self* (August 1991): 91.

Ganske, Mary Garner. "Take 2 to 10 Years Off Your Face." *Longevity* (May 1991): 62–64, 66.

Goldstein, Ross, M.D. "Strategies for Mastering Midlife: How to Win the Aging Game." *Bottom Line*. vol. 12, no. 14 (July 30, 1991): 5.

Griffin, Katherine. "Body Fat: How Much Is Too Much?" *Hippocrates*. vol. 3, no. 4 (July/August 1989): 92–94.

Hanson, Sherry Ballou. "The Fitness Alphabet." *Lear's* (September 1991): 54, 56–57.

Hatfield, Frederick C., Ph.D. "The No. 1 Sign of Aging — Wrinkles." *Muscle & Fitness* (February 1990): 234.

Levey, Gail A. "The Right Way to Eat Fats." *Parade Magazine* (November 10, 1991): 5.

Liebman, Bonnie. "The HDL/Triglycerides Trap." *Nutrition Action*. vol. 17, no. 7 (September 1990): 5.

Liounis, Audrey. "What Is Fat?" *First*. vol. 3, no. 39 (September 30, 1991): 32–33.

Loupe, Diane. "Prescription to Find a Good Doctor." *Atlanta Journal & Constitution* (October 29, 1991): C6.

Murray, Michael T., M.D. "The Natural Approach to Varicose Veins." *Health World*. vol. 4, no. 4 (July/August 1990): 37-38.

Otis, Carol L., M.D., and Roger Goldingay. "Exercise Abuse." *Shape*. vol. 2, no. 2 (October 1991): 90, 92–93.

Rae, Stephen. "Wrapping Up the Human Package." *Modern Maturity* (June/July 1991): 72–76, 91, 94.

Rozen, Leah. "Insomnia." *Self* (August 1991): 115, 141–42.

Shinkle, Florence. "To Lose Weight, Exercise 30 Minutes for 5 Days at Regular Rate." *Marietta Daily Journal* (November 1, 1991): 1E.

Spilner, Maggie. "We're Dancing!" *Prevention*. vol. 43, no. 12 (December 1991): 94–99.

Stuart, Eileen M., and Carol Wells, R.N. "Mental Powers." *Longevity* (November 1991): 26, 28.

"Treat Obesity as Addiction, Scientists Say." *Atlanta Journal & Constitution* (October 30, 1991): C5.

Weinhouse, Beth. "Your Health." *Redbook*. vol. 178, no. 1 (November 1991): 32.

Williams, Gordon. "Flaming Out on the Job." *Modern Maturity*. vol. 34, no. 5 (October/November 1991): 26–29.

Yudofsky, Stuart, M.D., Robert E. Hales, M.D., and Tom Ferguson, M.D. "Attacking Anxiety." *Longevity* (April 1991): 72.

PAMPHLETS

Breast Augmentation. The American Society of Plastic and Reconstructive Surgeons, Inc., 1988.

"Choosing a Qualified Surgeon." In *Guide to Aesthetic Plastic Surgery*. The American Society for Aesthetic Plastic Surgery, 1991.

Collagen Replacement Therapy. Collagen Biomedical, 1991.

The Decision Is Yours. The American Cancer Society, Inc., 1977.

M.D. Formulations. Herald Pharmacal, Inc., 1991.

The Most Often Asked Questions About Smoking, Tobacco, and Health and . . . The Answers. The American Cancer Society, Inc., 1989.

The Smoke Around You — The Risks of Involuntary Smoke. The American Cancer Society, Inc., 1987.

Tick, Tick, Tick. The American Cancer Society, Inc., 1990.

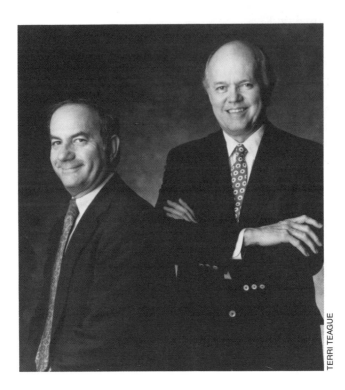

TERRI TEAGUE

Melvin L. Elson, M.D., is a diplomate of the American Board of Dermatology and a fellow of the American Academy of Dermatology, the American Society of Dermatologic Surgery, and the International Society for Dermatologic Surgery. An expert in the fields of preventive dermatology and soft-tissue augmentation, he practices at the Dermatology Center in Nashville.

John H. Hartley, Jr., M.D., is a diplomate of the American Board of Plastic Surgery, a fellow of the American College of Surgeons, and a member of the American Society of Plastic and Reconstructive Surgeons and the American Society for Aesthetic Plastic Surgery. Practicing at the Atlanta Aesthetic Surgery Center, he is renowned for his work in facial profiles and body contours.

Elizabeth Addison is the editor of *Cosmetic Quarterly* magazine and a partner in the Atlanta-based firm Communiqué, Inc.